DR TONY McCLELLAND

Staying alive
after 35!

The bare essentials

tfm Publishing Limited
Castle Hill Barns
Harley
Nr Shrewsbury
SY5 6LX
UK.

Tel: +44 (0)1952 510061; Fax: +44 (0)1952 510192
E-mail: nikki@tfmpublishing.co.uk; Web site: www.tfmpublishing.co.uk

Design and layout: Nikki Bramhill
Cover photograph: Sav Schulman, Auckland, New Zealand

ISBN 1 903378 27 3
© 2004 Dr T McClelland

Printed by Ebenezer Baylis & Son Ltd., The Trinity Press, London Road, Worcester, WR5 2JH, UK.

Tel: +44 (0)1905 357979; Fax: +44 (0)1905 354919.

Contents

Acknowledgements

The author wishes to thank his long-suffering wife and family for putting up with him during this project.

He wishes to thank all those friends who have offered inspiration and advice and, in particular, Dr. Ian Rosen for confirming the sheer brilliance and effectiveness of the McClelland dietary program.

Last but not least, he would like to thank his publisher Nikki Bramhill for her faith and unstinting support.

Dedicated to my lovely wife Bev,

Stuart, John

and

all my overseas family

Medical disclaimer

TERMS OF USE

The instructions and advice in this book are in no way intended as a substitute for individual and specific medical advice. They are not intended as a substitute for individual medical counselling. The information should be used only in conjunction with the guidance and care of your physician. Consult with your physician before adopting any program or treatment discussed in this book. This includes the dietary programs. Your physician should be aware of all the medical conditions you may have, as well as all medications and supplements that you may be taking. Patients with any long-standing medical condition should only proceed with changes to their diet and any other treatment, under direct medical supervision. Some of the recommendations will clearly be contra-indicated in certain subgroups. For example, patients on dialysis, patients on nitrates, and pregnant and nursing women, would clearly not be candidates for some of the recommended therapies or any of the dietary programs. Patients with severe kidney disease should rely only on specific medical advice from their doctors, and not use any of the advice in this book without the approval of their physician. Although every attempt has been made to keep the information in the book as current and accurate as possible, it should be recognised that medical knowledge changes rapidly and becomes rapidly dated. Under no circumstances shall the author or any other party involved in creating this book, be liable for any direct, indirect, incidental, special or consequential damages, including third party damages, that result from mistakes, omissions or other inaccuracies in the book.

IT IS EMPHASISED AGAIN THAT THIS BOOK IS INTENDED FOR INFORMATIONAL PURPOSES ONLY. THE INFORMATION IS WITHOUT WARRANTY OF ANY KIND AND SHOULD NOT BE USED WITHOUT THE EXPRESS CONSENT OF YOUR PHYSICIAN.

Introduction

At last, at last, some semblance of the truth at last

The idea for this book arose after many years in specialist medical practice. Like most of the rest of us, I am frequently lazy, often eat too much, have been known to drink far too much on occasion, and have neither the time nor the inclination for a routine structured exercise program. I have spent years giving advice on diet, exercise, and managing emotional stress. This has largely involved the promotion of the standard *schpiel* found in the self-help/health section of your local bookshop (you know, just after the "Why relationships fail" section and pretty close to the New Age area). With a touch of maturity, and the loss of the medical missionary zeal of the young and inexperienced (thank God), I came to realise that adopting the advice given required the self-sacrifice of a saint, the prissiness of an aged Victorian spinster, and the discretionary time of a pensioner. A predisposition to masochism would also be a bonus.

I have become more of a realist. I now give advice with which normal everyday people are likely to comply. I use drug therapy sensibly, focusing on the safest and most effective medications in the most practical formulations possible. I promote simplicity. This facilitates adherence. I have grown up. There is no doubt that appropriate modern medical therapy works. Having said that, a prescription for long-term drug treatment is almost never what people want to hear. They want quick fixes. Simple solutions, preferably with a New Age bias. And I would love to provide that. Honestly. Particularly because the market is huge. But I find I can't. I have seriously contemplated the issue, going as far as eating the tiny misshapen tomatoes that grow in a boggy patch around my father-in-law's state-of-the-art organic pit toilet. And that's at Xmas with a straight face. OK, I'll admit I was drunk at the time. Believe me, alcoholic premedication in industrial doses was essential.

You want a book with amazing and unsubstantiated claims about a single natural (or unnatural) product that solves a million of life's little emotional and physical problems, written by a guru, who was probably born in the Bronx but has since gone to great lengths to conceal the fact, then put this book back on the shelf immediately. Go find your book. There are literally thousands of such books in the health/self-help section, all written and marketed with you in mind. And as a result, your guru is probably now a millionaire, drinks industrial quantities of Moet, smokes 40 a day and has found herself a delightful and inexhaustible toyboy.

Still there? OK, back to modern medicines. Yeah, most of them really work. I mean, how boring is that? Particularly when you feel well and are too young to realise that life is finite. We can debate forever whether life is long or short, but believe me, it is finite. We aren't going to live forever. In our twenties and thirties when we are busy with career and family, that most useful of human defence mechanisms, namely denial, makes this hard to accept. Sure, we understand concepts of disease and death intellectually, but not at an emotional level during these decades. In our forties and fifties time seems to accelerate and all those precious sacrifices we made at work and such-like become a little less relevant. Furthermore, health starts to crumble (even if it is just the start of a second chin and an expanding waistline), and slowly but surely we realise that mortality is a long-term possibility. Our kids are usually adolescent at this stage and invariably think we are stupid, shallow, blinkered and mean (especially with the clothing allowance). And we start getting diseases. Not necessarily diseases that cause symptoms, but diseases such as high blood pressure and elevated blood fats that kill us nevertheless if untreated. So we try the transcendental meditation, seaweed extract, the herbal remedy with the unintelligible Latin name, and similar preparations. Sooner or later the natural supplements are rejected by some of us because they don't work. The remainder trundle on taking such treatment, feeling like a million dollars while high blood pressure and fats corrode their blood vessels, damage their hearts and kidneys, erode their brains, and ultimately cause overt catastrophe. Those of us who consult with our doctor are given drug therapy. More often than not however, treatment is inadequate, because the patient doesn't really want to take a "chemical". The doctor is thus pressurised not to prescribe appropriate doses or the multiple drugs that are often necessary to control these conditions adequately, or doesn't deal sensibly with unacceptable side-effects by modifying treatment accordingly, leading to non-compliance. And dare I say it? Sometimes the doctor just isn't up-to-date, which is hardly surprising given the volume of new medical information published every year. These issues continue to fascinate me. We could do so much better. A large percentage of patients with chronic medical conditions, who would benefit both in terms of survival and quality adjusted life years (QALYs - the magical years of your life when your physical and emotional health is optimal, and life is without a doubt worth living), are either on no treatment, or treatment that is sub-optimal by best practice standards. It is important to note that I am referring here to patients in developed economies who have medical insurance and absolutely no limitations in terms of access to first world medical care. One aim of this book is to provide patients with the basic knowledge sufficient to treat them to a long and healthy life by demanding the best care, without long-term starvation or physical deprivation. After all, life should be fun as far as possible, even for us Calvinists out there. And the meek, but only if that is OK for everyone else.

Modern man is an evolutionary masterpiece designed to survive wide variations in availability of food resources. We are built to endure prolonged famine, to feast during the good times, and to generally avoid any unnecessary exercise, such as walking instead of driving to the corner store. We are energy conservers by nature. We invent and cherish labour-saving devices. We have brains programmed to find sustenance and feast thereon. Our acute senses of taste and smell have been exploited by the food industry to seduce us further in these times of plenty (this is not a criticism but an observation). Portions have increased dramatically in size over the last 20 years, and the fat content (of fast foods in particular) exploited to save money and increase customer satisfaction. Fat food tastes good and satisfies. One super combo of fast food provides 80-90% of a child's daily calorie requirements. Sodas are now dispensed in 600ml and 1-litre bottles. This increases the calorie count dramatically. Studies in children have shown that this high volume liquid calorie intake has little effect in reducing feelings of hunger. Marketing of these larger volume sodas is clearly a great way to increase sales volumes and profit in a saturated marketplace. Childhood obesity has now reached epidemic proportions in the western world and the problem continues to grow, as do the children. Direct advertising of fast foods to the childhood market has been highly effective in exacerbating the problem and is morally dubious given the limited ability of children to make informed and rational choices (not that we adults do much better). Provision of soda machines and unhealthy fast foods in schools has compounded the problem, particularly because they are so effective in generating extra school funding.

Furthermore, the western world has been exposed to continuous abundance for the last 50 years or so. This is unique in the entire human historical experience. Blame dramatic scientific advances in farming techniques. Basic foods are now relatively cheaper in the West than ever before. The advent of television and more recently the personal computer, have increased the opportunity for entertainment while sitting on your butt. Most western kids watch approximately 25 or so hours of television a week. Television viewing and PC/computer games use have had a major negative impact on time available for physical activity and, of course, the attraction of exercise when compared to these modern sedentary delights.

OK, so what's the bottom line? Pretty obvious isn't it? No, the world is not shrinking. We are actually enlarging. Sixty-three percent of American and English adults are either overweight or obese. This is double the number a generation ago, when to be frank, fat people were hardly uncommon. In spite of this, we are living longer. We are getting fatter, and apparently unhealthier, and yet are living longer. This is largely the result of the quality treatments now available for most common medical conditions. Preventive therapy, however, could have a much greater impact than is currently the case, simply because it is not prescribed as widely and adequately as it should be.

Disease patterns are changing too. Living longer has its trade-offs. Forty percent of octogenarians have significant cognitive impairment i.e. dementia. Glory, glory, what a hell of a way to die: in a rest home, with a vocabulary of seven and double incontinence, while your 60 years plus children squabble over the will. OK. So we need strategies to minimise the risk of Alzheimer's disease and other causes of dementia.

Depression robs us of years both in quality and quantity. Recognition and appropriate therapy can change lives. And then all those other diseases like osteoporosis, breast cancer, prostate cancer, and unbearable in-laws. This book will enable you to understand the common life-threatening diseases, to avoid them as far as possible, and to have fun along the way.

Why don't we list the common causes of death or long-term disability (the dreaded diseases) in OECD countries in descending order of frequency?

1. Ischaemic heart disease (causes heart attacks and heart failure).
2. Cerebrovascular disease (strokes and such-like).
3. Chronic bronchitis and emphysema.
4. Lung cancer.
5. Pneumonia and other infections.
6. Neuropsychiatric disorders such as dementia.
7. Road traffic accidents and violence.
8. Unipolar depression/suicide.
9. Diabetes mellitus.
10. Gastrointestinal cancer (in particular colorectal cancer).
11. Breast cancer.
12. Prostate cancer.

> **The above is the list of diseases that are out to get us,**
> **that don't fight fair, and that will eventually kill or**
> **disable 95% of us unless we take sensible precautions.**

Take a close look, ladies and gentlemen. These are the major threats to a long and happy life. They are real. They are life-threatening conditions. They do not respond to rational debate or political correctness and, amazingly enough, are not prevented by treatments that don't work.

It is important to recognise that these diseases are not mutually exclusive. Seventy percent of deaths in developed countries are due to heart disease and stroke, but a range of other diseases and risk factors predispose to these illnesses. Most patients with diabetes, for example, die from heart attack or stroke. Obesity predisposes to heart attack, stroke and diabetes.

> **Importantly, heart attacks and strokes are not less common in females. They just manifest a few years later in the fairer sex, but cause just as much disease and disability in women as they do in men.**

Cancer remains the monster it always was, although the risks of the various cancers vary with gender. Depressive illness robs many people of decades of quality existence, and is thus a major cause of long-term disability. This condition is more common in women and remains a major cause of long-term, unnecessary anguish and suffering. People with long-standing illness are more likely to become depressed. Smokers are predisposed to heart attack, stroke, emphysema, and a variety of cancers.

So at this stage of the book, I have two choices. One is to wear the alternative New Age hat and waffle on about the wonders of ragweed thistle or mussel extract, focus entirely on this for the next few hundred pages, quote studies that wouldn't stand up to scrutiny by a preschooler, and flog the book. While doing market research prior to writing this book, I was informed by several publishers that this approach is the only guarantee of success in the self-help/health arena. Bull%^&* baffles brains, I was told (and that comment came from a very distinguished, successful and widely regarded female publisher!). Go for it. You can never overestimate the gullibility of the public. You will sell millions. We acknowledge that you are not photogenic, but you will be amazed how much we can achieve with computer graphics these days.

But I am not going to follow that route. Even with the best of intentions, it would be unethical (pity, but there is nothing worse than an overly punitive conscience). Anyway, as mentioned earlier, there is a huge market out there to deal with that type of publication already. But by God it is tempting. For the next few years however, I prefer to keep my soul intact. OK, call me insufferably self-righteous, but I am going to take the road less travelled. Maybe I can make a difference. Comments from one publisher suggest that it is likely to be a very, very, very small difference. But the public deserves better. So here we go.

There are a few issues that I would like to clarify before we go further. I have always been passionate about empowering patients (particularly women, who don't always get their fair share of health care), and encouraging them to involve themselves as far as possible in the management of their health. A recent article by the American Medical Association emphasised that the medical profession has not been particularly effective in promoting disease prevention. The focus of modern medical training is on treatment rather than prevention of disease. The public remains poorly informed and deserves better.

This book is fact-packed and contains the best quality medical advice currently available for the above listed diseases. The book may not look large but don't expect to assimilate everything discussed in a single gulp. The book is as much a detailed reference manual as it is a three-hour read. Feel free to take it along to your medical appointments. Most of the diseases addressed are complex. A simplistic and one-size-fits-all solution would be absurd. Having said that, as mentioned previously, most health and self-help books focus on simple issues and quick wins. They sell. They focus on one or two solutions to solve rocket science sized problems. They appeal because they promise that a one-hour read will provide you with a guarantee of eternal life, the meaning of human existence, and a perfect solution to everything in-between. But sadly, they commonly exploit and fail to live up to rigorous scrutiny.

I have used humour simply because it is part of my personal consulting style. It helps establish relationships and improve morale. I obviously do not use humour in situations where it would be inappropriate, emotionally insensitive or offensive to do so. Please do not misconstrue this as trivialisation of the diseases discussed. They are not trivial. They are after all, the major threats to human physical and emotional well-being in the new millennium. I grew up in a highly dysfunctional racist society, was drafted as a young doctor into an army fighting bitterly to maintain the status quo, and have spent the rest of my career in the frontline of medical practice. I have seen enough death and suffering (much of it preventable) to fill ten lifetimes. Humour is a sanity preserver for me. Therefore, if I do come across as flippant at times, I apologise in advance. It is not the intention.

Humour and absurdity are part of the human condition. We are all subject to foibles and oddities that are part of being human. I am just as vulnerable to these as the next person. I am an awful hypochondriac. I get a headache; I think I have a brain tumour. Influenza? I think I have meningitis. My wife get chills and a fever and I ask her if she can pick up the kids and a six pack of beers on her way home from work (ladies, have you noticed how much more susceptible men seem to be to the more severe strains of colds and influenza). If some of my comments in the book appear too caustic or ironic they are not due to special insight or superior scientific knowledge. They are simply there to inform, and provide an opportunity to reflect on how and why we make particular choices. There is no malice intended.

The clinical vignettes are based on real patients but occupation and location have been changed to preserve anonymity. I have tried to mimimise the use of incomprehensible medical jargon. However, as the book involves a summing-up of detailed medical research this is not always easy. I have included a summary box of the important points at the end of some of the more complex chapters. There is also a short practical glossary of medical terms, not covered in detail in the text, at the end of the book. And by the way, if you find some chapters (such as the statistics chapter) difficult to understand at first, don't worry. About 90% of us doctors are totally clueless when it comes to statistics, which explains the strange advice patients not infrequently receive.

One of the concerns about the ability of this book to reach the audience it so critically informs, is that it is too mainstream, and advocates conventional medical care in the bland old way. You know, middle-of-the-road, middle-aged and boring. Therein lies the tragedy. It is accurate, valid and scientifically the state-of-the-art. To emphasise again the points of a few pages ago, it lacks sensationalist, sometimes morally suspect, and controversial fashion of the month therapy that sells. For example, if you want to sell a book about AIDS, the most effective strategy to generate controversy and hence big sales, is to allege that the HIV virus is not responsible for the disease, or alternatively to come up with some half-baked theory about how you were cured using a mixture of lavender and crushed rhubarb stems. Of course there are MDs who recognise that patients are vulnerable to magic bullet solutions to health problems.

Similarly, some complementary and alternative practitioners also learn pretty early how to milk the market. So "the one magic bullet" is the name of their marketing game. Scientific medicine deserves better representation and access in the health section of any bookshop. I might be over the top occasionally, but what you learn from reading this should change the way you think forever. Even if it is challenging and goes against your philosophy of "wellness", you need to recognise the importance of the medical information contained. The book focuses on avoiding and treating the big killers of the new millennium. If that is not a relevant read we have a "denial" problem.

Classes of evidence

Grades or classes of evidence are used in an attempt to measure the quality of scientific research. They are mentioned in the statistics chapter, but as a summary, the following applies:

- **Class I** Well researched and definitely valid, usually based on one or more randomised controlled studies.
- **Class II** Research methods less precise and hence at greater risk of bias than Class I evidence, but still likely to be valid. Class II is often broken down into subclasses depending on how the research has been structured from a statistical point of view.
- **Class III** Expert opinion. This evidence is really only used when no reliable high quality research has been undertaken.
- **Class IV** Some systems do have up to Class IV evidence depending on their grading systems. There is no Class V evidence. Class V evidence equates to what grandma overhead at the bowls club.

Classes of evidence become less reliable from Class I to III. The use of evidence, and the evaluation of the quality of such evidence in medical decision-making, forms the basis of Evidence-based Medicine (EBM). The use of EBM has, to a large extent, transformed the practice of medicine from the old approach of umm, what shall we call it? Opinion? Best Guess? Thumb-sucking? Now there are several systems used to grade the quality of medical evidence. Importantly, all the systems tend to have a similar approach and all use the same basic underlying principles, although the grades or classes are sometimes structured differently.

I have no axe to grind regarding complementary and alternative therapies. It would be arrogant to assume that conventional medicine is the font of all knowledge regarding the human condition. If a product has no proven scientific value as a physical treatment but dramatically improves spiritual and emotional well-being, then as far as I am concerned that may well be good enough for the treatment of a specific symptom set. I have tried to provide you with some ideas on how to distinguish between valued treatments, treatments that have not been proven, and overt quackery. My intention is not to discredit alternative therapies *per se*. Nevertheless, most of these treatments will undoubtedly require rebranding in the next 50 years as increasing scientific scrutiny is inevitable, and evidence for most of these therapies as mainline treatment for serious disease is likely to be found wanting.

With all the angst and tragedy in life, a step backwards is occasionally necessary to provide a broader perspective. So now that we have been introduced, let's confront the obstacles to attaining long-term health and happiness together, with a lightness of step and an overriding sense of fun and optimism, as well as a large bag of tricks to minimise the risk of tragedy that day-to-day life can conceal.

As promised the advice given should require no insane or unrealistic physical or emotional sacrifice. The reason is that such advice seldom works in the long-term. I tried years ago to treat my body as a temple. It worked for about a month, after which time the demolishers moved in. I wasn't terribly keen to die earlier than I needed to, however. Fortunately there are painless, non-self flagellating, New Age free ways of achieving a long and healthy life using modern medicine. I know this might not sound cool but as mentioned previously, most modern treatments actually work.

This book has been written to promote optimal health for the average human living in the real world. Thus by definition, this is not primarily a diet or exercise manual. It informs and recommends the power of modern medical knowledge and technology to create a healthy internal physiological and psychological environment i.e. to make and keep you healthier. Knowledge empowers you to identify the best treatments and demand them. You may not look as healthy as a young Raquel Welch or Nicole Kidman at the end of the book, but in the long-term your body should be in better shape if treatment is indicated. Having said that, of course, we all want the one perfect long-term painless dietary solution, so as to look outrageously sexy or at least passable in subdued lighting. Therefore, this book will discuss diet and weight in some detail.

Given the dramatic breakthroughs in the treatment of most of the major potentially lethal diseases to which *Homo sapiens* is exposed, the failure to use such treatments as widely and effectively as possible is a tragic failure. Why is this so?

The answers are complex, but there is no doubt that the current purely scientific approach to the treatment of disease has failed the public badly. Human beings are not machines that require the odd lube and fine-tuning, the occasional widget replacement and regular service. They are spiritual and emotional beings with multiple drives and needs, varying prejudices, beliefs and philosophies. Paradoxically, the selection of medical students focuses on excellence in the physical sciences, with the unfortunate consequence that we focus on diseases purely as scientific challenges. Patients are essentially regarded as the substrate of our endeavours. To put it another way, an illness is regarded as a mathematics problem and a diagnostic challenge. The patient is that irritating woman that keeps trying to distract us as we strive for the scientific solution to this exciting problem. There are no really reliable tests to choose doctors on the basis of emotional intelligence or empathy. In addition, the natural "greenie" lifestyle is now seen as the route to mental and physical wellbeing. It is hardly surprising that there has been widespread desertion of the patient population to alternative therapies. Yet a wide range of recently developed preventive treatments have been shown unequivocally to improve the quality and quantity of human life. And easily! Without major lifestyle sacrifices! And that really works, even if recommended by a white-coated nerd who smells of formalin. Fortunately, the profession is attracting larger numbers of women than in previous decades, which can only be an advantage when it comes to representing the human face of medicine.

If you are a saint, a salvation army major, an athletic pensioner or a masochist, please put the book back on the shelf immediately. The content will not satisfy any of your basic needs. Get out there and punish yourselves. For the rest of you, please purchase the book immediately (I need the money. Also, my mother-in-law said it would never sell) and read on. The hidden wonders of modern medical technology are about to be revealed. A holistic understanding of what this can do for you, both physically and emotionally, should precipitate an informed discussion with your doctor regarding the various preventive therapies that may work for you. And make sure you're heard.

Both conventional medicine and complementary and alternative therapies could use a few home truths spelt out before we get too involved in strategies to help you live long and well, so let's get it over with.

References

1. WONG MD *et al*. Contribution of major diseases to disparity in mortality. *NEJM* 2002; 347: 1585-92.

2. Mortality by cause for eight regions of the world: Global Burden of Disease Study. *The Lancet* 1997; 349: 1269-1276.

3. MURRAY CJL, LOPEZ AD. Regional patterns of disability-free life expectancy and disability-adjusted life expectancy: Global Burden of Disease Study. *The Lancet* 1997; 349: 1347-52.

4. MURRAY CJL, LOPEZ AD. Global mortality, disability, and the contribution of risk factors: Global Burden of Disease Study. *The Lancet* 1997; 349: 1436-42.

5. MURRAY CJL, LOPEZ AD. Alternative projections of mortality and disability by cause 1990-2020: Global Burden of Disease Study. *The Lancet* 1997; 349: 1498-1504.

6. MOLD JW *et al*. Evidence-based medicine meets goal-directed health care. *Fam Med* 2003; 35(5): 360-4.

7. GUPTA M. A critical appraisal of evidence-based medicine: some ethical considerations. *J Eval Clin Pract* 2003; 9(2): 111-21.

Chapter 1

Alternative therapy, medical science and all that jazz

An alternative substance or supplement that is not harmful or illegal and makes you feel good is usually OK, provided that:

♦ You know precisely what it contains and the doses of the various constituents;

♦ You have no significant medical illnesses that it might aggravate;

♦ You are taking no other medications;

♦ It has a registered manufacturer;

♦ You don't overdose on the stuff (too much vitamin A for example is poisonous);

♦ A registered practitioner of some sort supervises the therapy (just in case litigation or some other form of accountability, is necessary).

Faith in a therapy is good. All medical studies have placebo groups. These individuals take a pill that has no effect at all. Nevertheless, about a third of this group feel better on therapy. Call it blind faith or whatever. It seems to work, at least in the short-term. Some alternative medicines have components that have been shown to be of scientific benefit. Blanket discounting of such therapy is therefore inappropriate. After all, one hundred million Americans can't be wrong (OK, I admit that's slightly tongue in cheek). Besides, many doctors have tried a variety of alternative therapies. Why do we find these so-called alternative options intrinsically so attractive? My theory of why this is so, is partially based on the survival advantage secondary to genetic selection. Until 70 years ago I'm pretty sure that doctors killed far more patients than they cured. It makes sense when one considers the therapeutic options then regarded as standard. These included bleeding the anaemic with rusty reusables, giving arsenic to the infected, using a variety of other noxious chemicals, purges and enemas, operating in last week's underwear, and doing all this in a totally insanitary environment. No wonder that much of the population had such a healthy distrust of the profession. Those poor individuals who had faith in the state-of-the-art therapies of those times not uncommonly experienced unsatisfactory outcomes (such as untimely death).

That segment of the population who intrinsically distrusted so-called modern medical breakthroughs, who preferred the application of raw meat as a poultice, herbs as folk remedies, and the use of a range of other options including various tractions and manipulations, didn't do so badly in comparison. This perhaps gave these individuals a genetic survival advantage. The net result is that a large segment of the population is genetically wired to be inherently suspicious of conventional medicine, and continues to harbour a distrust of modern, purely scientific methods of medical care. As mentioned earlier, white-coated, introverted, emotionally distant doctor-scientists have hardly strengthened the case for modern medicine. Medicine will always be an art that requires a sound scientific basis. The art has been overshadowed by modern technological interventions. Patients and the profession are poorer as a result. Furthermore, there are components to the art of healing which have been poorly researched by standard western medicine. These include the natural, spiritual and even sensory inputs available through complementary medicine. It is clear that some of these are innate and instinctive needs that are currently poorly satisfied by scientific therapies alone. The expectations of users of alternative therapies differ too. Because they use emotional reasoning, intuition and instinct when selecting such therapies, they are less demanding in their expectations of such therapy. If the aromatherapy or milk thistle doesn't make them feel better they move on. They don't have the rigorous expectations that they might for a medical procedure and do not sue if there is no perceived benefit. The positive outcomes they anticipate are more likely to be emotional, sensual, intuitive or spiritual.

When choosing a conventional medical treatment however, the expectations are based on more rational and less instinctive perceptions, the anticipated outcomes are more clearly measurable, and the contract is far better defined. All this has totally confused the medical profession, who are currently running around like headless chickens wondering what the hell to do about complementary and alternative medicine (CAM). There is huge and growing demand for CAM. This is occurring despite the fact that the burden of proof for most of these therapies is seriously lacking if well designed scientific studies are the accepted measure of effectiveness, yet the providers of complementary and alternative treatments are laughing all the way to the bank. Litigation insurance is negligible and there is minimal public demand for evidence that the treatments work. Attempts are being made by some medical faculties to narrow the great divide between conventional and alternative treatments, but this is obviously a retrogressive step from the scientific point of view.

Medicine requires a purely scientific research model to move forward in developing valid new treatments. The alternative approach is the anathema of modern medical research. Many alternative treatments rely at most on ill-defined qualitative measures of efficacy and will never accept the medical model. And why should they? Scientific research is extremely unlikely to demonstrate a true benefit for the vast majority of alternative interventions. Besides they are doing very nicely thank you. Not having a medical model, they can focus on the art of care, which medicine has lost. Their approach is reminiscent of the medical profession of a century ago. They alleviate symptoms (emotional, spiritual and physical) and comfort always. True cure, to put it mildly, remains highly controversial for most of such therapies. But then again, a century ago, modern medicine could cure practically nothing. One more thing, and it's a biggie. Greed, litigation, medical progress and suchlike have sent medical costs spiralling into the stratosphere. Alternative therapy is cheaper. So, for all those minor illnesses that would have gotten better without any therapy anyway, the medical profession is commonly no longer the first port of call. Damn.

So where to from here? The answer is obvious. Doctors are going to be forced to dramatically improve their practice of the art of medicine. Their technical skills are already being subjected to audit and are under increasing pressure to satisfy best medical practice. Relearning the art is a totally different story and will undoubtedly require more rigorous selection criteria to choose doctors who can relate to people. Amazing concept. The reintroduction of humanities, ethics, and interpersonal skills training into the medical curriculum is long overdue. A more balanced representation of gender and race in the profession is essential to resurrect the art of medicine. The indignity of procedures such as a rectal examination would be better understood by medical students if they themselves were subjected to a few of these procedures during training, perhaps even with a ward rounding group of doctors looking on. And what about those funny little gowns that patients are compelled to wear? You know the ones I mean. They open at the back and come only in one size, namely 10% too small. No matter what you do to try and conceal it, a portion of your butt will always be visible when wearing these. It would be nice to see a few surgical professors being compelled to wear similar gowns for a week of hospital work. And that's without anything underneath. Trust me, design patterns would change overnight. What do you mean shocking, doc? We subject our patients to these humiliations daily without a second thought.

Another area where we keep relearning the lessons of history is in the field of science. Is there any relationship between science and morality? Of course not. They are not even distant cousins. Science involves study and research into a wide range of subjects. It is neither a moral nor immoral concept and has no ethical connotations. Science can be used to benefit the planet, or alternatively exploited for other reasons. Yet scientists, including doctors, continue to regard their skills and experience as some kind of moral prerogative. I am not even going to go the Nazi Germany route. After all, that was over half a century ago and we are all so much more ethical now. Really? Pick an impoverished country in Sub-Saharan Africa. Shouldn't be hard. They are all impoverished. And the real beauty is that most have an annual per capita expenditure on health in the ten-dollar ballpark. So there are all these great diseases like HIV that can be researched using populations that have no access to state-of-the-art therapy. To be honest, they can't afford any treatment at all, so they are scientifically uncontaminated. This means we can nip into one of these countries and do a top-notch scientific trial on a new HIV drug, for example. One of the groups will get our new drug and the other (the placebo group) will get a cunningly disguised sugar capsule. After a year or two, we check the outcomes of the study. Then we pack our bags and our new drug, and wave goodbye to both groups involved in the study. No follow-up required. This is Africa remember. So much easier than to do expensive studies in a first world country where we would have a moral obligation to provide both groups with current best treatment and then add our drug. Furthermore, we would also be expected to follow these patients' progress in the long-term. We can't just dump them. Africa is so much easier and simpler to justify morally, because for Africans, no long-term treatment is affordable.

Can you spot the serious moral flaw in this argument? And is it just a hypothetical ethical question? No, this is how some recent research on treatment for HIV was conducted. Yes, by the caring profession.

And when it comes to money, doctors are at the least as greedy and corruptible as the rest of the population. I have worked in plenty of places where access to the private market is effectively controlled by cartels that claim to be the guardians of medical standards and patient safety, but who are infinitely more concerned about limiting competition and lining their own pockets. So when I talk about the ethics of alternative providers using unproven therapies, it needs to be seen in the context that conventional medicine has long lost the moral high ground. The days when professions at large were exclusively responsible for self-audit are over, and the faster we move forward in the direction of accountability to society at large the better.

Medicine also needs to become more affordable. We all know about Health Maintenance Organisations and so on, but the increasing medical demands of a rapidly expanding population of baby boomers with high expectations are not going to go away. Those countries with unrealistic approaches to medical litigation (such as no win, no fee), and outrageous settlement awards, will need to address these issues sooner rather than later.

And where to for alternative therapies 50 years from now? It is unlikely that most will stand up to rigorous scrutiny as cures of readily defined physical diseases. For many, a rational hypothesis of how they work does not exist. That's a bad start. The public, of course, is unlikely to become less demanding and less litigious, especially with all those law schools around. Most alternative therapies will simply have to rebrand themselves as components of the so-called "wellness" programs currently marketed to the financially flush, "worried well" middle classes of the western world. The reality of course, is that many of these therapies are identifying and exploiting this market already.

Alternative medicine is not a single entity and encompasses a wide range of different therapeutic options. The evaluation of alternative therapy as a single concept is thus simplistic and unreasonable. Alternative therapies include chiropractic, osteopathy, herbal remedies, aromatherapy, naturopathy (including phytotherapy and hydrotherapy), acupuncture, hypnosis, homeopathy, massage and nutritional supplements. Nevertheless there is a concerning lack of class I and II evidence for most of these therapies. What I am trying to say is that there is totally inadequate high quality scientific research available, and this makes recommendations on the use of these treatments difficult to validate. What is worth emphasising is the absence of any reasonably acceptable scientific theory as to how many of these treatments might work. This is where science is important, folks. The reality is that objective evidence as to whether a particular medication works requires rigorous scientific research.

Now I know what you're thinking. Here we go. Just another jealous doctor insisting on trials for treatments that have clearly helped me. Actually I have no major problems with the use of hands-on treatment for many minor or straightforward indications. I have personally had chiropractic treatment for low back pain. Studies regarding backache suggest that any form of treatment has the same outcome as any other treatment after a month or so, but chiropractic adjustment made me feel good. I would suggest that it is reasonable to use any form of non-ingested therapy for strains and muscular tension if it helps. Clearly the use of aromatherapy, chiropractic or homeopathy for the treatment of a heart attack would be worrying. As I said, these treatments almost certainly have their best value as part of a wellness program. They make you feel good, capitalism is God, and who am I to criticise about how you spend your buck. Nevertheless, be very, very careful about using these options for the big killers listed earlier in the book. It is just too risky in my view. This applies also to orally ingested supplements and herbal remedies, about which I will elaborate shortly. Having said that, I acknowledge again the intrinsic attractiveness of some of these therapies for many patients. Many modern medicines have been derived from plants, fungi, and bacteria, so the differences between alternative therapies and some modern medicines (for example, aspirin, digoxin, cocaine, penicillin) are not that extreme, at least in theory. Furthermore, middle class Americans spend as much on alternative therapies as conventional treatments. Should you feel strongly about using alternative therapy, please notify your doctor so that adjustments or monitoring of conventional therapy can be undertaken if necessary. And recognise their predominant value in providing sensual, emotional and spiritual well-being.

Does orally available alternative therapy (complementary medicine) have any intrinsic therapeutic activity? Are there products in the complementary sector, which really work beyond a simple placebo effect? If so, how do we recognize them? The short answer is we don't know. There are undoubtedly herbal and other products that have chemically active ingredients. Some have been shown to have effects that certainly could be effective treatments for a range of illnesses, at least in theory.

A well-known example is the use of St. John's Wort for the treatment of depression. There is class II evidence that supports the use of this agent in the treatment of mild to moderate depression. There is some evidence that the active ingredient may exert its therapeutic effect in the same way as selective serotonin re-uptake inhibitors (see chapter on depression). The agent thus contains an active drug. Why do some patients prefer to take St. John's Wort rather than a traditional antidepressant? Well, firstly it sounds like a natural non-medical treatment. People shy away from drug therapy for mental illness if they can, because of the perception that these drugs are mind-altering and addictive. In addition, the use of conventional antidepressants stigmatizes the patient as mentally ill. The conventional antidepressant also needs a prescription. So, you say, why the hell not use St. John's Wort? Well, because there is a downside. The FDA does not register St. John's Wort as a drug. "Natural supplements" and herbal remedies are not classified as drugs and are thus not subject to the scrutiny required to ensure consistency in manufacture or dosage. The purchaser has no idea of dosage or content. This can vary dramatically from formulation to formulation. So what? Well St. John's Wort contains at least one active medication that can interact with a range of other drugs. This can result in dangerous and even life-threatening drug interactions. Furthermore, the dose of the active ingredient can fluctuate significantly as the stringent FDA requirements are unnecessary. This is a pity because St. John's Wort is one of the alternative therapies that really seems to have something going for it in terms of efficacy. Remember too that serious depressive illness can be fatal, so inadequate therapy in this situation can have extreme implications. In short-term trials, side-effects were mild but did include indigestion, dizziness, allergy, headache, sexual dysfunction, increased skin sensitivity to sunlight and fatigue.

Gingko-leaf extracts are popularly advocated for the treatment of Alzheimer's and similar dementias, tinnitus (persistent ringing in the ears), poor circulation and nervous symptoms. They contain a variety of chemicals including terpenoids and flavonoids. Studies of efficacy using Gingko have had mixed results. We are not sure whether it works. It is not innocuous and can cause side-effects including headache, nausea, diarrhoea and allergic reactions.

Hawthorn extracts have been advocated for mild heart failure. If you have mild heart failure, make sure you are on your doctor's recommended drugs and avoid this stuff because of the risk of drug side-effects. Conventional drugs undoubtedly improve life expectancy.

Preparations of saw palmetto (sabal fruit if you must know) have been used for mild benign prostatic hyperplasia. There is limited evidence of effectiveness but side-effects appear not to be a major problem. Conventional therapies are of course the option.

I have discussed only a very limited range of alternative products simply because these are the only products which have been subjected to reasonable scientific scrutiny in the form of randomized trials.

Other natural products have sometimes been creatively manufactured to supplement any placebo effect. "Natural" pain relievers have, on occasion, been found to contain conventional analgesics such as anti-inflammatory drugs and paracetemol. Herbal teas and a variety of enemas have contained material that is potentially toxic. More recently, low doses of sildenafil (Viagra) have been detected in "natural products" for the treatment of impotence. The list goes on and on. The real issue is the absence of any consistency of manufacture, evidence of efficacy as therapy, and detailed information of dosage and content.

Remember too that there are plenty of "snake-oil" salesmen out there, and also undoubtedly, large numbers of substances that are unlikely to have any benefit beyond a placebo effect. I am the first to admit that these are often very effectively marketed. They appeal to physical and psychic needs in an emotionally, and spiritually, satisfying way. A natural herb extract to enhance libido is called "horny goat weed" extract. Is that a great marketing name or what? In my next life I am going to come back as an early 1970s San Francisco Ad person. Just imagine. You get to work at 11a.m. They feed you Moet champagne and seriously good weed. At about 3.00p.m. you start giggling hysterically and dreaming up product names. The competition wouldn't stand a chance. I reckon that some of these herbal supplements have marketing names that cannot fail to press our buttons. They know the essence of human weakness only too well. I am very, very, very impressed. Imagine a herb for impotence with the scientific name "flaccid thistle". It would stay on the shelf forever. I guess the mission statements of some of the failed dotcom start-ups were probably created using a similar approach.

Of course, the trade names used by the drug industry are also creatively designed. The difference is that they have been subjected to scientific scrutiny and proven to work. As a result, they tend to sell, irrespective of name. Extensive preliminary research, and ongoing audit, ensure the safety of such products. Furthermore, if you have an unacceptable side-effect the company is accountable. Imagine the difficulty in obtaining compensation for the nightmarish adverse effects of thalidomide if it had been a single component in a range of formulations marketed as pregnancy supplements. Marketing a product as a health supplement rather than a drug enables manufacturers to avoid the stringent FDA requirements essential for formal drug registration. This remains a legal loophole that will almost certainly be closed in the medium-term future. Recently, scandal erupted in Australia as a result of identification of failures in the manufacturing processes of alternative products by an Australian supplier of dietary supplements, leading to a range of adverse consequences for patients. This resulted in the recall of virtually all their alternative products, and serves to highlight the hazards of current loopholes in legislation of production and marketing of such agents.

Maintaining a sensible perspective is important, however. Alternative therapies vary widely and given the public support for such therapies, it would be naive and arrogant for conventional medicine to discount all such therapies out of hand. Further research will undoubtedly contribute to clarification of the role of individual treatments.

It is important to note that information available on the Internet regarding alternative products is frequently of very poor quality. A recent study in *The American Journal of Medicine* researched Internet information available for St. Johns Wort and rated the information available as being of a generally low standard.

- Complementary and alternative therapies (CAM) should not be dismissed out of hand.
- We cannot evaluate the validity of such therapy because we have limited evidence to verify the value of many of these treatments.
- Maybe conventional medicine is asking the wrong questions and, accordingly, providing the wrong answers.
- CAM is perhaps of best value as part of a wellness program.

References

1. DE SMET PAGM. Herbal Remedies. *NEJM* 2002; 347: 2046-2056.
2. SHEKELLE PG. What role for chiropractic in health care? *NEJM* 1998; 339: 1074-1075.
3. BODANE C, BROWNSON K. The growing acceptance of complementary and alternative medicine. *Health Care Manag (Frederick)* 2002; 20(3): 11-21.
4. OSTERMAN T, BEER AM, MATTHIESSEN PF. Evaluation of Inpatient Naturopathic Treatment - The Blankenstein Model. *Forsch Komplementarmed Klass Natuurheilkd* 2002; 9(5): 269-76.
5. BREUNER CC. Complementary medicine in pediatrics: A review of acupuncture, homeopathy, massage, and chiropractic therapies. *Curr Probl Pediatr Adolesc Health Care* 2002; 32(10): 353-84.
6. OPATRNY L. The healing touch. *Ann Intern Med* 2002; 137(12): 1003.
7. EISENBERG DM *et al.* Credentialling complementary and alternative medical providers. *Ann Intern Med* 2002; 17; 137(12): 965-73.
8. RADUSKI G. *Posit Living* 1999; 8(6): 16, 55.
9. MARTIN-FACKLAM M *et al.* Quality markers of drug information on the Internet: An evaluation of sites about St. Johns Wort. *The American Journal of Medicine* 2002; 113(9): 740-745.
10. MOYAD MA. Dietary supplements and other alternative medicines for erectile dysfunction. What do I tell my patients? *Urol Clin North Am* 2002; 29(1): 11-22.

Chapter 2

The truth about diet and health

Okay, so we are all getting bigger and wider. A marked reduction in energy expenditure coupled with increased dietary intake has resulted in these inevitable consequences. Clearly the appropriate response is to eat less, to eat sensibly, and to exercise more. This appears to be highly appropriate advice. But is it practical and is there good evidence that it is widely effective in the medium to long-term? The simple answer is NO! In fact, there is excellent evidence to the contrary. Of all individuals embarking on a diet, approximately half will have lost weight within three months. That figure drops to 5% or so at a year. Most of these dieters will in fact weigh more a year later than they did at the start of the diet. Sustained, effective weight loss is extremely difficult (as if you didn't know). Lecturing on health and longevity by focusing purely on diet and exercise simply doesn't work well for most of us in the long-term. Our genes, lifestyles, labour-saving devices, limited discretionary time, and environment of enduring abundance, conspire against the best efforts of almost all of us to maintain ideal body weight.

You don't need to be a rocket scientist to recognize this. Look around the health and diet section of any bookstore. Books on diet and exercise abound. If any single book provided the long-term dietary Holy Grail, the number of dietary options would dwindle dramatically. The diets themselves are often fascinating. Many provide strict limitations on the type of foodstuff that can be consumed. Thus, there are diets that minimise fat intake (standard scientific medical dogma); diets that minimize carbohydrate but allow unlimited fat and protein; high protein, low fat, low carbohydrate diets; diets restricted to grapes, grapefruit or any other fruit/vegetable; vegetarian diets; "organ-cleansing" diets of varying descriptions; drinker's diets; teetotaler's diets; diets requiring the consumption of industrial quantities of water daily; diets for the full range of religious dominations; and diets that promote brain, brawn or sexual organ growth and/or prowess.

New Age diets have become increasingly popular. The Internet provides a wide range of options. I was particularly fascinated by the hunter-gatherer diet. As you know, in prehistoric times, *Homo sapiens* survived essentially by moving from place to place, following animal migration for meat, and gathering wild flora for the vegetarian option. A few aboriginal people still live in this way. I worked as a doctor amongst the Bushmen of Namibia in Africa some 20 years ago. Believe me, the real hunter-gatherer life is bereft of pleasure. It comprises endless hunting or scrounging for food. Infant and childhood mortality is high and average life expectancy is about 38. Obesity is seldom a problem. Emaciation during the slim times (if you will pardon the expression) is universal among members of a tribe. So even though the term sounds kind of cool in a new age sort of way, the real life version sucks. And in the West we do have an equivalent. We call them bag ladies. Presumably the Gulag and seriously third world diets are out there in cyberspace, but being less politically correct and spiritually satisfying, are not widely subscribed.

Wow! By using the full range of options we would be one seriously disturbed species. Most of these diets quote high short-term success rates. I will explain in later chapters why this is so. I should also mention that some recommended diets have been well researched and are based on high quality scientific evidence. These are easier to spot as they seldom make outrageous claims and focus on long-term dietary strategies rather than quick fixes. The American or other Heart Foundations often recommends such books. My point however, is that long-term adherence to such diets is low because of the inherent difficulties and sacrifices required for compliance. The conspiracies of genes and all the goodies of the modern world consistently thwart success. As mentioned earlier, sustained success rates are about 5%. Excuse the pun, but the proof of the pudding is in the eating. I rest my case.

So should we call off the contest, head for the nearest fast food outlet with a wobble in the waist, and indulge in the nutritional delights of processed calorie concentrate? Ideally not, even if they will upgrade you to the super-duper triple combo, with eight pounds of chips, a megaton burger, and eight pints of soda for a mere 20 cents more. Why?

Because excess mass is not only a definite cosmetic disadvantage, but also a disease, which predisposes the victim to a range of other illnesses. These other illnesses spend their time trying to kill you. They are currently known collectively as the Metabolic Syndrome (the previous term was Syndrome X but then the cardiologists stole it for a totally different disorder. Nevertheless, you may find the term Syndrome X still in use as a synonym for the Metabolic Syndrome). There is no doubt that litigation versus fast food and soda companies that target children and schools in marketing campaigns, and continue to dish up such excessive calorie concentrates without appropriate health warnings, won't be too long in coming.

The metabolic syndrome predisposes practically every organ in the body to disease. The risks of acquiring this condition are both genetic and lifestyle related. Excess body weight produces a number of changes in the body's internal control mechanisms, as well as requiring a change of wardrobe. It is important to have some understanding of the mechanisms involved and the consequences, so that sensible decisions can be made about the appropriate responses. So read on fearlessly because solutions will be revealed as our tale evolves.

References

1. LEBOVITZ HE. The relationship between obesity and the metabolic syndrome. *Int J Clin Pract Suppl* 2003; 134: 18-27.
2. NESTEL P. Metabolic syndrome: multiple candidate genes, multiple environmental factors - multiple syndromes. *Int J Clin Pract Suppl* 2003; 134: 3-9.
3. BACHA F *et al.* Obesity, regional fat distribution, and syndrome x obese black versus white adolescents: race differences in diabetogenic and atherogenic risk factors. *J Clin Endocrinol Metab* 2003; 88(6): 2534-40.

Chapter 3

Metabolism gone mad

How does the body respond to excess weight, apart from the owner's pathetic attempts at concealment by wearing loose, longitudinally striped and/or dark clothing? The old bod has a genetic memory spanning millennia and is relishing this time of abundance. Time to store energy in preparation for the next plague or famine, it thinks. This of course, is deeply disappointing to the body's owner, who is neither anticipating famine nor wishing to look like a warehouse. Anyway, the storage forms of energy include carbohydrate (glycogen) and fat (triglycerides and cholesterol in a variety of forms).

Excess calories are not stored as protein unfortunately. This to my mind is pretty tragic. Imagine being able to eat your way to the Ms. or Mr. Universe title. What was God thinking while he was designing the human body? And another thing, why facial hair in post-menopausal women? And acne? And impotence after excessive alcohol consumption? But I digress. Where were we? Ah yes, protein. Protein is not primarily used for energy storage but can be broken down in times of food shortage to produce energy by a process known as gluconeogenesis (sorry folks, incomprehensible medical jargon does slip through once in a while).

The body can store about 5kg of energy as complex carbohydrate i.e. glycogen. Glycogen consists of large molecules made up of building blocks of glucose (the simplest sugar) and water.

The bulk of energy available is stored as fat however, usually in the least desirous places such as waist, buttocks, thighs etc., and, infuriatingly, never in the breasts if you are a flat-chested lady. Fat is also stored in the viscera (liver, bowel, omentum, heart etc). This explains the limitations of liposuction. Vast quantities of untapped fat lie submerged beneath the abdominal muscles. Furthermore, fat is an infuriatingly efficient way to store energy. One gram of fat contains three times the energy of a similar quantity of protein or carbohydrate. Excess body fat, and in particular visceral fat, increases the resistance of some organs to insulin. Detailed biochemical explanations are unnecessary, except to say that insulin requirements are increased in some body organs but not in others. The body must produce more insulin to cope as a result. Insulin is vital to promote glucose conversion to glycogen, the absorption of glucose by most cells in the body, the appropriate storage of fat, and the prevention of protein breakdown into sugar. Insulin enhances growth in some organs and in excess amounts can create problems in non-insulin resistant organs. For example, high blood insulin levels promote arterial muscle cell growth and fluid retention, both of which predispose to high blood pressure. As weight gain progresses, a vicious cycle occurs. With worsening obesity, the body is unable to increase insulin production sufficiently to cope with increased demand in some tissues and provides too much insulin for the needs of other tissues. Consequently, a full-blown metabolic syndrome may manifest. All this really means is that the body's internal chemical balance gets seriously out of kilter.

OK, enough of the gobbledegook. What are the features of the metabolic syndrome?

The list includes the following:

1. Excess body weight or obesity.
2. Increasing insulin resistance.
3. High blood fats with ratios that increase the risk for atherosclerosis (potentially causing a heart attack or stroke).
4. Prediabetes (a kind of half-way house) or overt diabetes mellitus. Diabetes has additional risks, including nerve, eye and kidney disease.
5. High blood pressure.
6. Increased risk of heart disease or stroke.

7.   Snoring and sleep problems that can culminate in sleep apnoea (and divorce).

8.   Fatty liver, which in some cases can lead to chronic liver disease.

9.   Arthritic problems including gout, and osteoarthritis of weight-bearing joints due to prolonged mechanical stress.

10. Polycystic ovarian syndrome.

11. And last but not least, unsightly stretchmarks.

I know what you're thinking. The b.....d has included every medical disease except warts, bubonic plague, acne and yellow fever. Well, not quite. What is particularly important however, is that the above list contains the conditions responsible for the overwhelming number of deaths (about 70%) in western populations.

With modern western medicine we can control most of these conditions very effectively.

As emphasised ad nauseam earlier in the book, we are becoming fatter and fatter, and more and more of us are succumbing to the metabolic syndrome and its rather nasty sequelae. This metabolic epidemic should be bumping us off in our fifties and sixties. Life expectancy should be decreasing dramatically.

Amazingly, this is not happening.

Westerners and those in other OECD countries are living longer and longer. For example, the average life expectancy for Japanese women is now 91, and for Japanese men, 83. Other OECD countries are not far behind. This is even more remarkable when one considers that life expectancy for males in the USA was only 47 in 1900. For females the figure was 52 years. When compared with those of normal body weight, obese individuals do have a reduced life expectancy (of about 8-12 years on average), but are still living considerably longer than their forefathers.

Can this be explained by improved plumbing, the death of Typhoid Mary, reduced alcohol consumption, increased consumption of seaweed extract, garlic and parsley, and camomile tea? The simple answer is no. Certainly in the first half of the 20th century, improvements in nutrition, management of infectious diseases, and sanitation had some impact. However, in the last 50 years most improvements can be ascribed to more effective prevention and treatment of the big killers, namely heart and vascular disease. And what is particularly amazing is that we do not do it particularly well. Many people receive care that is suboptimal according to the best evidence-based medical treatments. For example, only 60% of adults in the US who have both hypertension and health insurance (no causal relationship between the two exists, I promise) have their blood pressure treated to ideal targets. Treatment of diabetes is suboptimal in the vast majority of patients. It is only in recent years that doctors have started thinking laterally. Focusing on totally unrealistic dietary targets and lifestyle sacrifices inevitably produces little impact on the disease process (remember the 5% success rate for diet). We now have first class medical evidence that shows outcomes can be dramatically improved by aggressively treating other risk factors associated with diabetes and the metabolic syndrome. Given that at least 63% of us either have or are predisposed to the metabolic syndrome, let's look at the issues a little more closely.

- The so-called metabolic syndrome (or syndrome X) will probably be the major cause of disease and disability in this century in OECD countries.
- All the individual consequences of this syndrome are treatable or preventable.
- In spite of this, appropriate treatment is not provided to the majority of people who would clearly benefit from such therapy.
- The medical profession has failed to address health prevention issues adequately in the past.
- This makes it increasingly important for individuals to understand personal health needs and to demand that such needs are addressed.

References

1. CALLE EE *et al.* Overweight, obesity, and mortality from cancer in a prospectively studied cohort of US adults. *NEJM* 2003; 348(17): 1625-1631.

2. CARR MC. The emergence of the metabolic syndrome with menopause. *J Clin Endocrinol Metab* 2003; 88(6): 2404-11.

3. RUSSELL JC. Reduction and prevention of the cardiovascular sequelae of the insulin resistance syndrome. *Curr Drug Targets Cardiovasc Haematol Disord* 2001; 1(2): 107-20.

4. PARSONS PA. From the stress theory of aging to energetic and evolutionary expectations for longevity. *Biogerentology* 2003; 4(2): 63-73.

Chapter 4

Basic dietary principles

Why don't we examine the individual components of the metabolic syndrome to see how we can minimise the adverse effects on our poor innocent bodies who, after all, still think it is 50,000 BC.

Obesity is a biggie. I know, I know, I know that I promised this wasn't going to be yet another diet book. But there are some basic principles about diet that are important. These are not always accurately portrayed as such in the media. In addition, the big wide world of advertising not uncommonly makes outrageous or invalid claims to promote different products. It's a jungle out there. For example, there are "good" fats, "bad" fats, neutral fats and ratios which, if you buy the right margarine, practically guarantee a body like Nicole Kidman, ten cents off your next purchase of the same, and just possibly immortality. The same goes for red meat, white meat, etc.

So let's do the basics:-

Diet should be high in **fibre**. OK, I know everyone knows this. Eating half a kilogram of pure bran kills your enthusiasm for the chocolate and jelly pudding. This is the first advantage of fibre. It fills you up (not very satisfyingly in my personal experience, but better than nothing). It helps prevent constipation in a way that does not damage the colon. It prevents diverticulosis, a condition very common in western populations. Diverticula are thin outpouchings of bowel which can become infected or perforate. It is likely that fibre rich foods reduce the risk of colon cancer. Recent studies assessing pure fibre intake have admittedly failed to demonstrate a reduction in colon polyp and cancer rates. It may be that the deficiency in these studies was to focus on fibre *per se* instead of focusing on diets not purely high in simple fibre but rather on diets rich in fibre-containing foodstuffs such as fruits, vegetables, legumes, and whole and high-grain fibre products. In other words the fibre may be a surrogate marker for a variety of vitamins and nutrient constituents of fibre-containing foods that prevent the cancer. This suggests that natural fibre-containing foods are preferable to pure bran and proprietary bulk-forming preparations.

Fibre, including in particular, soluble fibre (viscous, and found in oats, peas, beans, and some fruits), is effective in lowering cholesterol and glucose levels. Recommended daily intake of fibre is in the region of 35 grams. Do your best folks but let's keep it simple. Even with compliance there is a downside. Undigested fibre is fermented by colonic bacteria to produce methane and a variety of other noxious gases, if you get my drift. This socially unfortunate consequence does tend to improve with continued fibre intake. Worse case scenario, you can blame it on the male sitting next to you, whose protestations of innocence are not only unlikely to be believed, but also regarded as extremely ungentlemanly. Of course, if you were trying to make a favourable impression on that particular male, you have a problem.

Low calorie fibre consumption is particularly useful as a filler. Leafy green vegetables, figs, celery, raw onion and cucumber contain practically no calories, and together with tomatoes and extra-virgin olive oil, are the essence of the famous lipid-lowering Mediterranean diet. Mediterranean-style seems to translate into a reduced risk of heart disease and stroke, particularly when accompanied by medicinal amounts of alcohol. Watch the quantity of olive oil though, girls. It is calorie rich. The diet sounds inherently sensible otherwise.

So much for fibre. I mean who really wants to live exclusively as a ruminant (except maybe cows and vegans). Now for dietary **fat**. This ubiquitous and tasty food component has given the human race (and in particular our arteries) more than a few problems. There are two major types of fat in the human body, namely **cholesterol** and **triglycerides**. Now to let you into a nasty little secret that the medical fraternity has long concealed from you guys. Are you sure you are ready? This may come as a shock. *Homo sapiens* is a mammal. There, I have said it. We are actually part of the animal kingdom (I personally found this difficult to accept until I saw my first Jerry Springer show). And one of the amazing things about mammals is that they can manufacture their own fat i.e. triglycerides and cholesterol.

What does this mean? Firstly, next time your doctor suggests that your cholesterol levels are excessively high, inform her that you synthesized all the cholesterol yourself. Especially if you are a vegan. Cholesterol is only found in animal products, mainly animal fat and egg yolk. This confirms that all the cholesterol in the blood of a vegan has been personally synthesized. That should wipe the smug expression off her face, because implicit in her observation is the suggestion that you have been pigging out. Secondly, our bodies tend to regulate fat levels within a certain range, which varies for different individuals. For example, if dietary cholesterol intake is reduced, then hepatic (liver) synthesis is increased to compensate. Does this mean that diet has no impact on serum cholesterol levels? No, because compensation is incomplete. Nevertheless, even scrupulous dietary reduction of cholesterol and saturated/non-liquid fat intake can only drop blood cholesterol levels by 10-15%. Therefore, if your normal cholesterol is more than 15% above ideal (and note I said ideal), then diet alone is not going to do it for you. Furthermore, most of us are well aware of the relationship between high cholesterol and heart disease and have made some dietary adjustments to address the issue. As a result, further attempts at dietary therapy alone often have minimal impact, demoralising both patient and doctor (the doctor less so if you carry health insurance).

Thus cholesterol (and triglyceride) levels are subject to a feedback control mechanism to maintain levels within a defined range. In some of us, the feedback mechanism is less than perfect and cholesterol is overproduced as a consequence, producing unacceptably high levels irrespective of diet. There is usually a genetic component to this. That's why some skinny athletes have a sky-high cholesterol level and the odd Sumo wrestler has the same levels as a starving vegetarian. Triglycerides are the principal storage form of fat and consist of three chains of fatty acids linked to glycerol. They appear less closely linked to heart disease than cholesterol but certainly play some role, particularly in subgroups such as diabetics, and should not be ignored. Both cholesterol and triglycerides are attached to protein carriers in the bloodstream to produce compounds called lipoproteins. The combination of carrier and fat can increase or decrease the risks for vascular and heart disease depending on chemical make-up. HDL (High Density Lipoprotein) contains some cholesterol but is a "good guy" i.e. the contained cholesterol has been extracted from the fatty (atheromatous) plaques that cause atherosclerosis. LDL (Low Density Lipoprotein) also contains some cholesterol. LDL is a real sonofab... It promotes the accumulation of fatty plaques. High triglyceride levels lower HDL levels and also contribute in other ways to fatty plaque formation.

OK enough already. What should we all be eating to reduce LDL cholesterol and triglyceride levels?

It's really easy according to the medical scientists, and that is why dietary therapy alone has such dismal results. Eat less saturated fat (animal fat found in steak, burgers, beef, bacon, lamb, eggs, cream, ice cream, English breakfasts, chocolate, cheese, pizza, cheese-cake, full cream milk, crème Brule and virtually all classy French food for example), and less refined carbohydrate (bread, sugar, jelly, cake, muffins, pancakes, syrup, American and Canadian breakfasts, cookies, chips etc.). Minimise consumption of trans-fatty acids. These are found in stick margarine, vegetable shortenings and deep fried foods. Margarine with a high content of trans-fatty acids tends to be solid and lard-like at room temperature but check the label. Trans-fatty acids increase LDL cholesterol levels.

Eat the good fats. The good fats include monounsaturated and nonhydrogenated polyunsaturated fats (also known as omega 6 fatty acids). Such fats are found in peanut, olive, soybean and rapeseed oils. Eat fatty fish at least twice a week (kind of hard if you live in the Sahara). Fatty fish and fish oils contain long-chain n-3 polyunsaturated fatty acids. These are better known as omega 3 fatty acids. They are also found in some plant oils including canola and flaxseed. Eating fatty fish twice a week, or taking fish oil supplements, has been shown to improve long-term survival following a heart attack. There is as yet no definite evidence that they prevent heart disease in healthy individuals, but risks do seem to be less in individuals at high risk, so providing you like fatty fish, it seems sensible to partake of this regularly. There is now a suggestion that eating fatty fish more than four times a week might be a bad idea, because of mercury accumulation in some fish species. All this tells me is that extremes are bad. Of course, Eskimos will probably just have to take their chances. The alternative natural option is about ten fish oil capsules a day.

This sounds very alternative and inherently more attractive than taking a "drug" to control high blood cholesterol levels. Unfortunately, there is a downside. You run the risk of smelling like pickled herring. Reflux of the oily material into the throat can also occur. I am not joking. Blind dates will gag at the first whiff. Unless you are planning to live in the Arctic Circle or marry a fishmonger, this supplement is best approached with caution. Fish oil eaters should also avoid swimming in shark-infested waters. Realistically, if we all adopted this advice we could probably kiss cold-water fish stocks goodbye within a decade. Stocks are already under pressure. And of course, there are six billion human beings on the planet. The demand would be environmentally catastrophic. Is this ever mentioned? Of course not. Who prefers a natural alternative? The marketeers know. Middle class, professional and educated people who are also environmentally aware. They prefer a "natural alternative" to a "medication" but not at the expense of decimating threatened species. So, of course, there would be serious consumer resistance to this particular product. There is nothing sadder than cynical manipulation of altruistic, well-meaning individuals who believe that they are making sensible and reasonable choices. Natural is not always better. The use of rhino horn, shark cartilage, and a range of other threatened natural resources is deeply concerning when considering the lack of evidence of benefit for these products, and the very real risk of ultimate extinction of species, such as the great white shark and the white rhinoceros. Sadly, the "alternative products" manufacturing business is fast losing its scruples in the hunt for profits.

Next, NO butter. Damn. Margarine sparingly, and only margarines practically devoid of trans-fatty acids, as emphasised above. These tend to be softer and easily spreadable. Proper low fat milk only. Cook ONLY with vegetable oils. Better still, boil or stew rather than grill or fry.

Reduce salt intake. Some medical scientists have suggested we avoid adding salt altogether. They reassure us that after two months or so, you can't tell the difference. Now is that practical or what? A bit like ordering a salmon and cream cheese bagel without the cream cheese and salmon. I am sure that after a few months we won't miss the salmon and cream cheese. But is the small reduction in blood pressure achievable, with this "user-friendly" regime, worth the misery and deprivation? Like I said, sometimes a tablet is not a bad option. Even the real hunter-gatherer or Gulag diet might be a soft option in relation to this, particularly if the salt-free diet is continued obsessively and in perpetuity.

Protein intake is recommended to be about a gram per kilogram (2.2 pounds) of body weight per day. Sources of animal protein should be predominantly in the form of white meat i.e. poultry and fatty fish, with red meat perhaps once or twice a week. Low fat dairy products are a good source of protein and calcium but the fat content should be checked to ensure the product is truly low in fat. Vegetable sources of protein include legumes, soya beans and nuts.

OK folks, take a step back and pause for breath. So now we know why dietary therapy is a bit of a nightmare. It remains a constant contest versus our genetic drive, it deprives us of the pleasure of eating sublime food, it makes us feel guilty and unworthy and, even worse, it fails as a long-term option for 95% of us. Do we deserve this? I think not.

With the super-duper fibre-containing foods we are all eating as part of our perfect diet, adequate nutritional intake of vitamins, essential minerals and other micronutrients, should be a cinch, right? Well, not necessarily. Calcium and vitamin supplementation (for example **group B** and **D vitamins**) have a role to play in maintaining health. For these reasons, daily supplementation is indicated. Vitamin D by supplement should be 800 I.U. daily. Additional **calcium** is important in patients at risk for osteoporosis, the vast majority of whom are female. Read all about it in the relevant chapter.

Excessive vitamin A consumption can cause vitamin A toxicity and supplementation is not recommended. Severe toxicity can be fatal. This was first described during a search for the Northwest Passage from Europe to the Dutch East Indies. Snowbound and starving sailors consumed polar bear liver and developed an acute severe illness secondary to vitamin A toxicity that was not uncommonly fatal. This has also been described in vitamin-obsessed individuals in the West who take industrial doses of multivitamins. Vitamin A deficiency practically never occurs, except in situations of extreme starvation. Minor excesses in vitamin A consumption have been recently shown to increase the risks for osteoporosis and fracture. It seems that vitamin A, in excessive amounts, stimulates the osteoclasts (cells that promote bone breakdown). So forget the vitamin A folks. Too much of a good thing can be bad for you after all (as if those of us who suffer from frequent hangovers didn't know this).

A very topical issue in the medical and lay media in the last decade has been research into free radicals and antioxidants. No, free radicals are not out of control university students with extreme left-wing views. Free radicals are toxic (for toxic read poisonous) by-products of a host of essential chemical reactions in the body. They are usually rapidly neutralized by a variety of antioxidants. Failure to promptly detoxify these agents can lead to serious tissue damage. Research on the adverse effects of free radicals in a wide range of conditions from stroke to premature aging continues. Because antioxidants rapidly eliminate these chemicals, an intrinsically plausible and attractive hypothesis has been proposed. This suggests that loading our bodies with antioxidants has got to be good for us. Even more attractive is the fact that so many naturally occurring antioxidants are available. These include vitamin C, vitamin E and beta-carotene. Preliminary research suggested that these agents might just reduce the risks of atherosclerosis (including heart attack and stroke) and delay aging. A gargantuan market has evolved to deal with this. Because these agents are "natural products", they are particularly attractive to the alternative and complementary markets.

Now for the evidence:-

Beta-carotene (a vegetable vitamin A precursor) is an antioxidant with purported cardio-protective properties. Class I studies have not confirmed this. Furthermore, there is some evidence to suggest that excessive beta-carotene might just increase the risk of cancer. Drop this supplement folks, unless you are fond of funny yellow skin discolouration. For more information on the quality grading of medical research, please refer to the chapter on statistics.

Vitamin C has received great acclaim in the last few decades. It prevents scurvy, a discovery that saved generations of sailors from suffering and death in the great days of sail. The vitamin functions as an antioxidant and cofactor in a range of essential biochemical synthetic processes in the body. Scurvy is potentially fatal and is only seen in prolonged severe deficiency. The illness has been documented in situations of gross nutritional neglect in the developed world (for example, isolated old widowers living on toast and tea for prolonged periods). Unfortunately, large doses of vitamin C do not prevent the common cold, heart disease and the range of other conditions for which the vitamin has been advocated. This is most regrettable for manufacturers of the product but is true. Class I evidence says so and that should be good enough for all of us. The vitamin is potentially toxic in large doses. Risks of overdose include an increase in the incidence of indigestion, diarrhoea, kidney stones, and possibly iron overload. Really, there has got to be a better way to spend your money in the search for perfect health, unless of course you are planning on becoming a 16th century sailor.

Vitamin E is an antioxidant and does a great amount of mopping up of toxic oxidants in animal models. As mentioned above, there are sound hypotheses as to why such agents might reduce the risk of atherosclerosis and hence heart attack and stroke. Several class I studies have shown no clinical benefit in humans. Furthermore, no clearly defined dietary vitamin E deficiency syndrome exists in humans. Much has been written about vitamin E and the self-help sections of most bookshops are filled with books of encyclopaedic proportions claiming vitamin E as a wonder drug. There is no good evidence to support this. It seems like our diet provides enough antioxidants already. In fact randomised studies investigating the role of such agents in the prevention of heart attack and stroke suggest a trend towards increased mortality in the groups allocated to treatment with vitamin C and vitamin E. There is class II evidence that large doses of Vitamin E (1000 units twice a day) may be helpful in slowing the progression of Alzheimer's disease, but the research has many potential biases. For the moment vitamin E is not a standard recommendation as a supplement. And don't even mention selenium or other antioxidant supplements. The lack of benefit of these agents has been well documented. What is more worrying is that some of these supplements in large doses are potentially harmful. For further information on the use of supplements visit the UK Food Standards Agency website at www.food.gov.uk/healthiereating/vitaminsminerals.

You realise of course, that I am digging my own grave (metaphorically speaking) by disclosing this information. Bland, boring, conventional scientific advice hardly ever sells in the self-help/alternative section of bookshops, and that's where the money is. If this book isn't published or fails to sell, I am planning to reinvent myself as an eastern mystic and self-help guru. After all, business is business. Having said that, I realise that it will not be easy. My wife tells me that I look like a real schmuck in a Kaftan, and we are not even Jewish.

The **B group** includes a range of vitamins including thiamine (vitamin B1), riboflavin (vitamin B2), niacin (vitamin B3), pyridoxine (vitamin B6), cyanocobalamin (vitamin B12) and folate (pteroylmonoglutamic acid, if you must know). These agents are water-soluble and storage capacity in the body is limited. They play a role in essential reactions involving protein synthesis, carbohydrate production and utilisation, and single carbon transfer reactions necessary for DNA synthesis.

Enough of the biochemistry. Give us the facts. Deficiencies of these vitamins are seen in the context of gross malnutrition coupled with increased demand. In the developed world, skid row is the place to go if you are seeking seriously vitamin B deficient individuals. High carbohydrate and alcohol intake, coupled with lack of vitamin B, can produce a range of illnesses that include Wernicke/Korsakoff syndrome, beri beri, peripheral nerve damage, glossitis (inflammation of the tongue), angular stomatitis (inflammation of the corners of the mouth), delirium, spinal cord damage and megaloblastic anaemia. Suffice to say, most of these conditions are pretty lousy and some are irreversible or fatal without prompt vitamin replacement. I bet you don't know anyone with any of these conditions. The reason is simple. Most people who buy books of this calibre have a diet sufficient to prevent significant vitamin B deficiency. We do know however, that these vitamins are not fat-soluble and cannot be stored in the body in large amounts. We also know that current recommendations regarding optimal daily requirements may be too low. We know that increasing daily folate, vitamin B6 and vitamin B12 intake, reduces blood homocysteine levels. Elevated homocysteine levels increase the risk for heart attack and stroke (see Chapter 12). Folate supplementation in pregnancy reduces the risk of cleft palate and spina bifida. Overdose of vitamin B compounds is rare because these agents are not fat-soluble, so storage facilities are limited. Anyone who has taken a vitamin B supplement will have noticed that a significant amount of any dose is promptly excreted in the urine. I do recommend supplementation. This should be sensible and not exceed 5mg of **folate** and two vitamin B complex tablets daily. Use a formulation recommended by your pharmacist. The real tragedy is that mandatory fortification of flour with folate should have been legislated years ago. This practice would almost certainly have saved tens of thousands of lives in the UK alone by reducing blood homocysteine levels and hence the incidence of heart disease and stroke.

Regarding trace elements, fluoride supplementation reduces dental caries. The amount contained in fluoride-containing toothpaste should be sufficient to satisfy dietary needs. Overdose can occur in adults. Mottled unsightly teeth are the obvious clinical manifestation. Supplementation of other essential trace elements including selenium, chromium, choline, copper, magnesium, zinc and manganese, is unnecessary in healthy individuals. Check out the UK Food Standards Agency website before considering taking any obscure supplements. Discuss the need for potassium and magnesium supplementation with your doctor if you are taking diuretics, are diabetic, or are suffering from any chronic gastrointestinal condition. Additional nutritional support may be necessary in these and other chronic illnesses. Save the rest of your money for something more emotionally gratifying.

References

1.   ANGELESCU I *et al.* Add-on combination and maintenance treatment: case series of five obese patients with different eating disorders. *J Clin Psychopharmacol* 2002; 22: 521-4.

2.   LIPS P. Editorial: Hypervitaminosis A and fractures. *NEJM* 2003; 348(4): 347-9.

3.   HU FB, WILLETT WC. Optimal diets for prevention of coronary artery disease. *JAMA* vol 288(20): 2569-78.

4.   YANCY WS *et al.* Diets and Clinical Coronary Events. *Circulation 2003*; 107: 10-16.

Chapter 5

Real diets for real people

No! That's not what I meant!
That dress definitely does not make you look fat.

OK, so this book is all about living longer, healthier lives without demanding unrealistically harsh and unworkable strategies. So how to approach dieting? Well, the previous chapter defines the broad principles.

Any diet chosen needs to be medically sound,
and to have both an initial program followed
by a long-term maintenance strategy.

Most diets found on the bookshelves or the Internet are effective in the first few weeks. There are several reasons for this. Weight loss in the first week or two is often dramatic. Wow, thinks the enthusiastic dieter, at this rate I will be the spitting image of Twiggy in a few months. The truth regarding early weight loss is another closely guarded medical secret in order not to discourage enthusiastic fat people from at least trying to lose weight. The first 5kg or so of lost weight is not fat at all. It comprises the body glycogen stores, located largely in the muscle and liver. Glycogen molecules, as mentioned previously, are large complex structures built from simple sugars (glucose) and water. Thus, in fact what is lost in those early, halcyon, and watch-out-world-here-comes-the-second-Twiggy days, is water and sugar. Damn.

Now the diet becomes less fun. Firstly, the body thinks it has just spent the last week in a concentration camp. Brace yourself for a famine, command those ancient genes. Body metabolism slows so less energy is consumed. The mobilisation of fat to provide energy occurs, but because fat is such an efficient compact form of calorie storage, small amounts provide substantial energy. A good example of this is the obvious effect when fat is thrown into a fire. The ensuing conflagration is almost equivalent to the effect of gasoline. Weight loss screeches to a dead stop, or at best a painful, drawn out process of milligram weekly losses. The diet, of course, almost invariably restricts overall calorie intake and often precludes the consumption of some normally essential component (such as fat or carbohydrate). Morale plummets. Adherence is hardly helped by the exclusion criteria of the said diet. And does your boyfriend / fiancé / husband / love, notice? You betcha, but only if weight loss has been dramatic. For the reasons described above, sustained dramatic changes in shape and weight are very difficult.

Then one morning you walk past a pastry shop. The aroma of fresh bread and pastry assails the senses. Break out time say the genes. The prognosis for this sustained famine is worrying. Get in there and eat, for God's sake. Such temptation can be resisted to a point, but for 95% of us genetic sanity prevails and we succumb. And that, Madame, is the thin edge of the wedge for the diet. Oh well, let's start again next Monday. Yeah right, say the genes. They don't call us the thrifty (energy-conserving) genotype for nothing.

Hey, isn't something missing? Human beings are satisfied for some hours after a big meal and are not perpetually hungry. We are well designed by and large (excuse the pun) except, unfortunately, for the new millennium. Perhaps I need to expand on this and explain some of the underlying mechanisms that regulate bodily functions in this regard.

A large number of so-called "negative feedback" loops exist to control production and secretion of hormones and other chemicals in the body. These loops function by providing feedback on the levels of the particular chemical so that production, and hence body content, can be continuously and appropriately adjusted according to need. There are a wide variety of triggers that stimulate appetite and in addition, triggers and chemicals that say. "No! Definitely not another ice cream!" The study of hunger mechanisms is currently undergoing extensive research (partly to look for the ultimate diet pill). A wide range of hormones and chemicals are currently being studied to evaluate their roles in appetite control.

A recently identified and currently topical chemical released in direct proportion to total body fat stores is called leptin. Leptin informs the appetite centres of the brain of body fat status and when enough is enough. There is an impression that individuals prone to easy weight gain have appetite centres less sensitive to leptin, and in some cases inadequate production of leptin. Another substance called ghrelin (what a ridiculous name - who the hell dreams these terms up?) is secreted by the stomach and has the opposite effect. Ghrelin stimulates appetite, commonly overriding conscious dietary self-control with consummate ease. Other chemicals that contribute to the dietary tango include insulin, pro-opiomelanocortin and pancreatic polypeptide. However, control of food intake has emotional, cerebral, gastrointestinal and biochemical components, is extremely complex and clearly still inadequately understood, so I won't ramble on any further regarding this.

What can we do to cheat our way out of obesity? Fighting weight gain is a lifelong marathon. As we age so our metabolic rates slow. This means less energy consumption to maintain basic body functions. The obvious consequence is easy, easy weight gain. This is why a 20 year old male can drink twelve cans of high calorie beer daily for a month without consequences, whereas a 65 year old female just has to walk past a deli to gain a kilogram. Weight loss definitely becomes more difficult with age.

I for one, however, am somewhat saddened in having to regard my lifetime journey as a dietary marathon. What about having fun and taking time to smell (and, if desperate, eat) the roses? Life is not a rehearsal. What about mimicking the hunter-gatherer routine i.e. simulating periods of feast and famine? This is also known as yo-yo dieting or weight cycling. Unfortunately, (or fortunately), extreme fluctuations in body weight do not seem to be healthy, can predispose to binge eating, and have been associated with overt bulimia, depression and possibly increased mortality. So let's forget the extremes folks. We are only human. Settle for a long-term, balanced dietary pattern. Sure, short-term aggressive dieting is often necessary, possibly with the help of the drugs discussed below. Large regular weight fluctuations are best avoided however.

What about the use of drugs to knock the weight off? There are a number of drugs used to treat obesity. Essentially they fall into two categories. One group suppresses appetite and the second group interferes with fat absorption. The combination of fenfluramine and phentermine (known as fen-phen) was widely used in the US for years. A rare side-effect (primary pulmonary hypertension and heart valve damage) developed in a small proportion of users. Because this condition is usually fatal, these and similar drugs are best avoided.

More recently, orlistat (trade name Xenical) has become available. This agent inhibits lipase, the main pancreatic enzyme responsible for fat digestion. When taken with a fatty meal, orlistat inhibits absorption of up to one third of dietary fat. The drug is mildly to moderately effective in the short-term. It is pricey. The real downside is occasional anal leakage of oily fat and staining of underwear. The drug should clearly never be used before a heavy date. The rather unpleasant side-effects do tend to modify behaviour, and consumption of the drug often leads to reduced fat intake. This drug does not prevent carbohydrate (sugar and starch) absorption.

Another new drug is sibutramine (an appetite suppressant that has not shown the adverse consequences of the earlier products in this class). Short-term use is worth considering after discussion with your doctor. Newer drugs such as topiramate are also undergoing evaluation but are not currently registered as dietary agents.

Is surgery an option? For morbidly obese people with a BMI in excess of 35, surgery should be seriously considered as a long-term solution to their problem. Morbid obesity takes years if not decades off life expectancy. There is a large body of evidence that confirms that obese individuals are prone to extensive discrimination even in today's politically correct environment. Obesity is associated with lower educational attainment, occupational success, median income, and increased risk of depressive illness. The surgical options vary and are not without risk, particularly because of the technical difficulties and risks of post-operative complications in this patient population. Laparoscopic (keyhole) surgical approaches are evolving and should be a welcome addition to the surgical armamentarium as techniques and equipment improve.

Now for the diets:-

Firstly, determine your target bodyweight. To do this you need to measure your body mass index (BMI). This is calculated by dividing your weight in kilograms by your height in metres squared. To make this easy, the best thing to do is to go to any of the large search engines on the Internet (for example Google) and type in the term BMI calculator. Bingo. A list of websites containing the relevant calculator appears. If you happen to live in a country that is non-metric, find a calculator that provides the relevant conversions for feet, inches and pounds. If your BMI is less than

18.5 you are underweight. The normal range for BMI is 18.5 to 24.9. A BMI from 25 to 29.9, implies that you are overweight. A BMI of 30 or more equals obesity.

We all need to recognise that most diets have an initiation phase followed by a maintenance phase. It is pretty pointless starting on the maintenance phase when the wedding is in three weeks and 6kg just have to go. Urgent requirements for weight loss are occasionally part of real life. As long as you don't make a habit of yo-yo dieting. Remember my concerns voiced a few paragraphs ago. Having said that, lapses are inevitable in life and using the techniques of initiation therapy for several weeks four or five times a year is unlikely to be harmful, particularly when compared to the health risks of long-term obesity. Anyway, let's deal with maintenance first:

♦   **Maintenance therapy** must provide balanced long-term nutrition. Most of you will be aware of the food pyramid regarded as the ideal formula for a balanced and healthy diet. The broad base of the pyramid includes unrefined, fibre-rich carbohydrates and vegetable sources of protein, moving up to the middle of the pyramid (low fat dairy products, white meats such as poultry, and oily fish), and finally reaching a very tiny tip of animal fat and cholesterol. This diet is widely supported by the medical community and recommended by the **American Heart Foundation**. This is a rational option for maintenance therapy. Recently, the increased intake of fatty fish and monounsaturated/omega 3 and omega 6-rich vegetable sources of fat (peanut, olive, canola oil etc.) have been emphasised as the critical part of the middle portion of the pyramid because of the favourable consequences in lowering cholesterol levels.

♦   This diet is far more likely to be effective if used with other individuals in similar circumstances. This is part of the reason that **Weight Watchers** works reasonably effectively. You are all in the same boat and peer pressure promotes adherence to the program (a bit like good old Alcoholics Anonymous).

♦   The cheapest, and at least as effective option, is the **Dr. McClelland** maintenance diet. This option has one serious drawback. It is simple and impossible to market effectively as a franchise. No one can capitalise on my maintenance diet. It will never make me rich. Apart from a daily vitamin and mineral or two, it recommends no special marketable supplements. All this is very sad.

♦ **Anyway, here is the McClelland diet.** Adopt those broad guidelines recommended above that are acceptable to you. Don't waste your time trying to adhere to a maintenance dietary program that you find intolerable. Long-term compliance will simply not happen.

Let me summarise again the basic dietary principles. Vegetables, fruits and whole grains (including high fibre bread and cereals) to provide fibre, carbohydrate and some protein. The omega 3 and omega 6 rich vegetable oils, and omega 3 rich fatty fish recommended provide most of the fat. Animal sources of protein to be largely derived from the fatty fish, low fat dairy products and poultry. Vitamin B complex, folate, vitamin D 800 I.U. and calcium one gram daily as supplements. You should be taking these anyway.

Then, simply decrease the size of all the portions. Yes, that's the secret! Fewer beans, less fish, far less potato on each plate. As a rough guide, start with a reduction of about a third in portion size. Maintain the balance in such a way that the diet retains its usual variety. The medical literature confirms that this does just as well in the long-term as any other recommended diet. Remember, we have all been eating monster portions for the last 20 years. You are not going to starve. I promise. The remarkable thing about my diet is that it actually saves money, as the requirement for essential supplements and the other necessities of commercial dietary programs, are practically non-existent. In fact, with reduced expenditure on food, the diet should save you even more. Some knowledge about the low calorie sources of food to satisfy the munchies (the desperate urge to sneak a snack between meals), is essential of course. These are described in two bullet points below. And remember, if you do sneak in a snack, deduct the equivalent caloric amount from your next regular meal.

♦ Perhaps the easiest way to reinforce the emphasis on smaller portions is to have smaller dinner plates. I admit this sounds ridiculous but hey, it might just keep you focused on sensible portion sizes. You think only the portions got bigger over the last 20 years? In order to compensate, the plates have too. Creative presentation of meals is sensible to make the meal look more substantial than it is, if only to satisfy the inappropriate expectations of the fast food generation.

♦ IMPORTANTLY, give yourself permission to cheat a few times a week. Do not order the celery delight at a top New York restaurant. When taken out to dinner have a ball. I call this the cheat technique. It works well because it is realistic. I first recommended it to adolescent diabetic patients. We are all going to cheat occasionally anyway. So remove the guilt. It is normal. Even our genes say so. An orlistat tablet might be an idea during these episodes.

♦ Remember again, that leafy green vegetables, cucumber, tomatoes, raw onion, and figs are good low calorie fillers during uncontrollable urges to cheat, cheat, cheat (well, what did you expect? An offer of a cream and jelly doughnut?). Other low calorie vegetables include asparagus, artichokes, spinach, broccoli, celery, red and green peppers, beetroot, radishes, carrots, turnips, watercress, zucchini and leeks. Grapefruit, nectarines, melons or apple skins are the lower calorie fruity option. If you can't face any more plant food, cheat by eating animal protein-containing products (fish, chicken, lean meat, low fat dairy). Dr. Mac's golden rule of the munchies is to avoid all breads (simply because they provide the perfect excuse for a sandwich), cereals, refined carbohydrates (i.e. any sugar-containing food), all types of nuts, and chocolate.

♦ Don't forget the advantages of Mediterranean-style cuisine.

♦ Herbs are extremely low in calories and add some excitement to almost any meal. Incidentally, oregano, sage, peppermint, garden thyme, lemon balm, clove, allspice and cinnamon are loaded with naturally occurring antioxidants. Other useful herbs include basil, mint, marjoram, rosemary, chives, garlic, parsley, fennel, dill, tarragon, lemon grass, curry leaves, sorrel and dandelion.

♦ Drinking eight glasses of water daily, is strongly recommended by the manufacturers of bottled water. What can I say? Great marketing is great marketing. The marketeers and manufacturers have followed a trend. Water is effective as a filler, particularly on a full stomach and especially following the consumption of high fibre grain and cereal products, as these tend to be water absorbent. So make a habit of having a glass or two of water from time to time and always at the end of any snack or meal in order to confuse those greedy genes into thinking you have eaten more than you actually have.

♦ There are four primary taste sensations, namely sweet, bitter, salty and sour. Sweet has been the real problem for the human race over the last few decades. I can see how the sensation provided a survival advantage in past millennia. How many poisonous substances are sweet? Practically none. How accessible are sweet foods in the hunter-gatherer's world? They are a rare and seasonal delicacy and consist of fruits packed with refined sugar. In ancient times these comprised an instant source of calories and energy and presumably had the same effect as sugar drinks have on 5 year olds today. Just imagine. After exposure to a treeful of pineapples, those with a sweet tooth were up and running, fighting, seducing and mating with anything in their path. Their genes were inevitably passed on, explaining much of current middle class behaviour. Naturally the human bliss associated with eating sweet, refined carbohydrate-rich foods has been maximised by the market. This is why low-fat, carbohydrate-rich diets have been such a failure. Amazingly enough, gradual reduction in intake of sweet tasting foodstuffs can, in the medium-term, eliminate the cravings for these foods. To be honest, any long-term dietary strategy is only going to be effective if you can modify your tastes, so that refined carbohydrates are no longer a significant part of your diet. Artificially sweetened soft drinks and calorie-free sweeteners in tea and coffee are acceptable for those with a sudden uncontrollable craving for something sugary. Gradually reduce the amount of artificial sweetener and in 3-6 months, the old bod will adapt. I promise.

♦ Go easy on the salt. For ethical reasons I have sneaked this in, hoping you might not notice. By the way, adding more vinegar to salad dishes is a useful way of masking the reduced salt content.

♦ If you are not controlling weight in spite of the adjustments, start the initiation program again and for subsequent maintenance, reduce carbohydrate portions to about half your pre-diet intake, rather than reducing protein.

♦ Still not working? Reduce carbohydrate intake further and focus exclusively on my favoured carbohydrate vegetables and fruits as the carbohydrate portion of your diet. And consider orlistat or sibutramine for a period. Remember, long-term dietary failure is almost invariably linked to excessive calorie intake from refined calorie-rich carbohydrates, those damned sugars and starches. Our genes find such foodstuffs exquisitely appealing and need to be bewitched, bothered and consistently seduced by alternate dietary options.

♦ Trust your scale. If you are not controlling your weight, dietary intake is excessive and needs downward adjustment.

And now for **initiation therapy**. It's three weeks before the wedding. You feel fat. In fact, to be perfectly honest, you are a bit fat. Panic time. Most starvation-type diets work well, but hell they are tough to adhere to.

♦ If you have no illnesses and really want to get the groom to see you at your skinny best (or vice versa), the Atkins diet induction program may be worth considering. It is effective for rapid weight loss in those prone to cheating, largely because it does not restrict protein and fat intake. Very little carbohydrate is permitted. **Dr. Atkins** was intelligent. His induction diet does allow very low calorie vegetables such as lettuce and cucumber, for example. As mentioned earlier, these are fibre and water-rich but contain virtually no calories. As described previously, your body quickly exhausts carbohydrate reserves. Fats are broken down for energy. Ketone bodies, one of the products of fat breakdown, contribute as an energy source but, more importantly, suppress appetite. And the diet is restrictive. Believe it or not, there is a limit to how much fat you can eat if that is all you confront day-in day-out. Take a double dose of multivitamin during this period. If really desperate, you might throw in an orlistat tablet, but be aware of the downside.

Widespread, mainstream medical support for the Atkins diet is variable, particularly for long-term maintenance therapy. The issues are controversial because of the relationship between high animal fat intake and heart disease, but the diet remains extremely popular. Reassuringly, a recent article in *The New England Journal of Medicine* confirmed that the Atkins diet is effective short-term (more effective than the low fat diet to which it was compared in the study) and seems to have no significant adverse sequelae. Blood fat profiles were actually improved in the Atkins group. Furthermore, diabetics and other patients with the metabolic syndrome were included in the study. Unfortunately after a year, there appeared to be no difference in outcomes between the two diets in terms of weight loss, and failure and drop-out rates for both diets were high. This is disturbing because any study environment is somewhat artificial when compared to the real world. Simply being involved in a study often motivates patients, resulting in considerably greater benefits than those seen in daily practice. But you and I know all about long-term success rates anyway. As I mentioned earlier in the book, a single magical diet does not exist. If you want more information about the Atkins diet, read the Atkins diet books.

♦ A second option is the **Weight Watchers** initiation program.

♦ The third option is the **McClelland** program. Here, individual carbohydrate portions are reduced to a maximum of one third of the previous size, and either orlistat or sibutramine or both (be warned, they are not cheap) taken, but only after discussion with your physician. Use my low calorie carbs listed in the maintenance section as the bulk of your carbohydrate intake. Maintain fish and poultry intake at two thirds of your pre-diet intake. Take the vitamins and calcium as mentioned in maintenance and use the other tricks of maintenance therapy as indicated. Remember my golden rule of the munchies. Aim at a target of about one kilogram (2.2 pounds) per week weight loss. Remember that weight loss is going to be slow as body glycogen reserves are exhausted, which means that greater sugar and starch (but not animal protein) restriction may be necessary if targets are not being met. The initiation program can be continued until target weight (based on BMI) is achieved, provided that regular liaison and close monitoring by a physician is part of the program if target weight requires more than 10kg of weight reduction. Monitoring of blood chemicals and vitamin levels may be necessary under these circumstances.

Did I hear someone mention the word **exercise**? Oh dear, here we go. Well, exercise is important for a multitude of reasons. It is less effective for weight loss than diet alone, given our madly efficient little fat cells, but certainly helps the process. How much exercise? The evidence suggests that 30 minutes of moderate exercise (brisk walking or jogging for example) five times a week significantly reduces cardiovascular morbidity and mortality. The benefit is likely to be linear so any physical activity is better than none. Exercise improves muscle strength, co-ordination, mental well-being and cardio-respiratory fitness. Isn't that just wonderful? The reality of course, is that 40-50% of adults hardly ever exercise. The reasons are multiple and related not only to sloth, as the exercise gurus and puritans would have us think. Time is a major factor. We exist for much of our lives with work and home obligations that are exhaustive and demanding. Our days are long. Living in northern Canada or Scotland is not exactly conducive to an evening winter jog, particularly at the end of a 12-hour day. We naturally all have periods during our lives where a regular exercise commitment is easy. School, college, pre-children and retirement, are the times that come to mind.

The large gap in the middle is an issue. Jogging became fashionable in the 70s. Prior to that, running for the hell of it was regarded as rather odd. There were no fitness or aerobic clubs in the 50s. Gyms were distinctive places; strictly men only and filled with the delicate aroma of rotten underwear and old sweat. Maybe 2% of men used such places, yet average body weight was considerably less than today. The figures are simple to explain. They are unrelated to disease or nutritional improvements. Food consumption has increased but is only part of the problem. The reality is that people used far more energy in the activities of daily living even 40 years ago. Cars, elevators, automatic toothbrushes, television, remote controls, PCs and computer games have markedly reduced daily energy expenditure. We drive 200 yards to the corner store. We transport kids everywhere. We take the elevator instead of the stairs. We have petrol lawn mowers with custom leather seats. We use golf carts instead of walking the course. OK, OK. I know I am starting to sound self-righteous. The point however, is this. For a long-term exercise program to be effective throughout all the phases of our lives, the simple things are important. Climb staircases, walk instead of drive (if it is practical - I don't mean from New York city to Phoenix, Arizona), and structure your everyday activities in such a way that some physical activity is a natural part of your routine. Also, play plenty of golf. If your spouse enquires why, show him this book. If you have the opportunity, by all means add aerobics, jogging and pumping iron. Remember though, that sustainability and avoidance of extremes are the cornerstones of any long-term, life-changing exercise program.

By the way, there is increasing evidence that obesity increases the risk for a range of cancers. These include cancers of the oesophagus (gullet), stomach, gallbladder, pancreas, kidneys, colon, and a variety of blood cancers. Gender specific cancers, more common in obese women, include cancer of the uterus, cervix and ovary, and prostate cancer in obese men. These increased cancer risks nevertheless represent a far lesser hazard than the risk of dying from the consequences of the metabolic syndrome in any individual patient.

- There must be a zillion diets out there.
- The implication is that no particular diet works for everyone and that most diets fail to be effective in the medium to long-term.
- Dietary therapy should have initiation and maintenance phases.
- Not all fat is bad for you. Healthy fats have no bad effects on total blood cholesterol and triglyceride levels and may improve them.
- Fat is very calorie rich however.
- Carbohydrates can also make you fat, and refined carbohydrates (like sodas, sugar and cookies) are packed with calories.
- Diet should be balanced with a focus on smaller portions of each item, particularly cholesterol, saturated fats and refined carbohydrate.
- Dietary options include the Atkins diet (for induction), Weight Watchers and my smaller portions diet.
- Exercise is highly desirable but programs need to be appropriate to competing time demands.
- Supplementation of some vitamins (but not others) is sensible.
- Medications are available to help if necessary.

P.S.

1) Avoid painfully thin, sanctimonious doctors and dieticians (or, if you are really tempted, beat them to death).

2) The information in the above chapters may not provide the specific recipes but contains all the essential information necessary for effective weight loss.

This information is in fact the state-of-the-art when it comes to advice about long-term safe and effective weight control. Treasure it and use it. It really does work!

References

1. PIROZZO S *et al.* Review. Advice on low fat diets is not better than other weight-reducing diets for sustained weight loss in obesity. *EBM* 2002 Nov/Dec: 175.
2. FONTAINE KR *et al.* Years of life lost due to obesity. *JAMA* 2003; 289(2): 187-193.
3. NIELSEN SJ, POPKIN BM. Patients and trends in food portion sizes, 1977-1998. *JAMA* 2003; 289(4): 450-453.
4. FOSTER GD *et al.* A Randomised Trial of a Low-Carbohydrate Diet for Obesity. *NEJM* 2003; 348(21): 2082-2090.
5. SAMAHA FF *et al.* A Low-Carbohydrate as Compared with a Low-Fat Diet in Severe Obesity. *NEJM* 2003; 348(21): 2074-2081.
6. DRAGLAND S *et al.* Several Culinary and Medicinal Herbs Are Important Sources of Dietary Antioxidants. *J Nutr* 2003; 133: 1286-1290.
7. CUMMINGS DE, FOSTER KE. Ghrelin-leptin Tango in Body-weight Regulation. *Gastroenterology* 2003; 124:1532-34.
8. LEUNG WY *et al.* Weight management and current options in pharmacotherapy: orlistat and subutramine. *Clin Ther* 2003; Jan; 25(1): 58-80.
9. ULLRICH A *et al.* Impact of carbohydrate and fat intake in weight-reducing efficacy of orlistat. *Aliment Pharmacol Ther* 2003; 17(8): 1007-13.
10. ROLLS BJ *et al.* Portion size of food affects energy intake in normal weight and overweight men and women. *Am J Clin Nutr* 2002; 76(6): 1207-3.
11. ATKINS RC. *Dr. Atkins' new diet revolution.* Avon books, New York, 2002.

Chapter 6

Bye-bye high blood fats

As mentioned in the previous chapter, diet and exercise have only a limited impact on blood cholesterol levels. Generations of patients have been brutalised (OK, I am exaggerating a little) into thinking that it was their fault. That is part of the fun of being a doctor. We can accuse patients who have been living on celery for a month that they have been cheating on their diet. The problem is compounded by the fact that early cholesterol-lowering agents were either ineffective or produced unacceptable side-effects or outcomes. One particular agent was found to be downright dangerous. The drug, clofibrate, did reduce triglyceride levels and did increase HDL (the good cholesterol-containing lipoprotein) levels modestly. This resulted in a reduction in heart attack and stroke. Unfortunately however, the study group showed an increase in overall mortality. Consider the scenario: "Mr/Ms. Patient, if you take my medication the good news is your blood fat levels will improve. Unfortunately, your overall life expectancy might be shortened." No wonder complementary remedies became an exciting alternative. Another major player, a drug called cholestyramine, was safer and more effective, but has to be consumed with meals and can cause abdominal discomfort and flatulence. Adherence to a drug that has to be taken three times a day for an asymptomatic condition creates issues. Although the flatulence tended to improve with time, compliance with therapy certainly didn't. Newer and safer fibrates (improvements on clofibrate) have become available over the last 20 years or so, and some (for example, gemfibrozil) have improved life expectancy in heart attack survivors.

By far the most important breakthrough in drug therapy of high cholesterol has been the development of statins. These drugs are HMG CoA (hydroxymethylglutaryl Coenzyme A) reductase inhibitors. No, you do not have to memorise that. They literally switch off cholesterol production.

The consequences for blood cholesterol levels have been dramatic. Overweight, sedentary middle-aged matrons are now able to waft around with blood cholesterol levels equivalent to those of preteen girls. Is this important? After all, uncomplicated high cholesterol is asymptomatic. Your blood cholesterol reading can be off the top of the scale and you can feel like a million dollars (and I mean US dollars, not Zimbabwean dollars). High blood cholesterol is simply high blood cholesterol. It is a predisposing factor to cardiovascular disease, in particular heart disease and stroke. These diseases don't play fair. They don't care if you have been using a foot balm, herbal tea, or some other therapy designed to support you from a placebo point of view. They fight dirty. They present with catastrophe, not uncommonly death or irreversible disability.

OK, I better elaborate. As mentioned previously, high blood cholesterol levels cause clogging up and hence narrowing of blood vessels. Blood vessels are the essential supply lines for oxygen and nutrients (the combustible energy sources essential for life). What are the consequences of sudden blockage of such vessels? A common presentation is sudden death. This tends to be dramatic and instantaneous, and for these reasons doesn't allow a hell of a lot of room for negotiation. About one third of patients with ischaemic heart disease (i.e. occluded cardiac blood supply) present in this way. Another third present with heart attacks. These patients present with sudden blockage of a vessel supplying part of the heart, but survive the attack with variable degrees of permanent heart damage. Many of the remainder present with angina. Angina occurs due to a transient insufficiency in blood flow to the heart muscle, without causing muscle death. Other presentations include irregular heart rhythms and failure of the heart muscle to function effectively leading to heart pump failure.

These multiple scenarios make one thing patently obvious. Prevention is better than cure. With modern drug therapy we can now offer painless prevention. I admit that swallowing a tablet doesn't sound intrinsically attractive. Most westerners inherently prefer the "natural options". As mentioned previously, early drug therapies were sometimes pretty dubious alternatives. We have moved on though, folks. Strongly supported by the legal fraternity (I admit, that's slightly tongue in cheek), we have been scrupulously careful to ensure that treatment is as safe and effective as possible, not only in reducing blood cholesterol and triglyceride levels, but also in improving quality of life and life expectancy. The statins have been demonstrably effective in improving life expectancy in groups at moderate and high-risk for ischaemic heart disease or stroke. Best evidence strongly favours the use of these agents in patients with a history of ischaemic heart disease and stroke, adult diabetics, and individuals with a family history of premature ischaemic heart disease i.e. heart disease below the age of 55, and a personal blood cholesterol level in excess of 4.5mmol/l, in spite of appropriate dietary therapy. It is likely that other subgroups will benefit from this therapy and that these guidelines are probably conservative. Certainly all asymptomatic individuals at significant risk for any vascular event (stroke, heart attack, angina or transient ischaemic attack), should strongly consider the use of these agents. It is becoming obvious that the most important factor to take into account when deciding whether to use statins is the patient's individual risk for atherosclerosis, rather than the actual blood fat levels.

Is there a downside? Of course. The drugs cost money. There is a very small risk of liver inflammation which occurs in a small proportion of users. This can be identified by monitoring liver function using serial blood tests, and is almost always reversible on cessation of therapy. Some patients develop muscle aches. These are usually dose-related and respond to dose reduction. A very small number of patients taking statins develop more significant muscle injury, particularly when they are used in combination with fibrate drugs (used to reduce triglycerides), but such combination therapy is seldom indicated. Available statins include atorvastatin, simvastatin, lovastatin, pravastatin and fluvastatin. Atorvastatin is the most potent agent and in addition, appears significantly more effective in lowering blood triglyceride than the other agents. A recent addition called cerivastatin was found to be associated with a higher than anticipated risk of muscle damage (rhabdomyolysis) in combination with fibrates and has been withdrawn. In spite of the above caveats, the risk-benefit ratio of these drugs in patients at moderate to high risk for cardiovascular disease strongly favours their use in the groups described above.

It is important to realise that this therapy is long-term. It reduces high blood cholesterol levels and protects against premature death in that way.

The benefits both in terms of cholesterol levels and life expectancy are seen early after onset of treatment in high-risk groups. Blood cholesterol rises to pre-treatment levels within 48 hours after cessation of therapy.

Right, folks, that's one for the sensible folks i.e. the rest of us.

- We make about 90% of our cholesterol and obtain only 10-15% from diet.
- Therefore, dietary modification seldom has a dramatic effect on blood cholesterol levels.
- Modern cholesterol-lowering medication prevents heart attack and stroke and should be regarded as essential for all at increased risk of these diseases.

References

1. BRAUNWALD E *et al*. *Principles of Internal Medicine*, 15th ed. McGraw-Hill, New York, 2001.
2. SCHUSTER H. Managing the high-risk patient: therapeutic approaches in 2002. *Atheroscler Suppl* 2003; Mar;4(1): 15-20.
3. NASH DT. Statins. Evidence of effectiveness in older patients. *Geriatrics* 2003; 58(5): 35-36, 39-42.

Chapter 7

High blood pressure - hypertension

You think fighting with patients about taking cholesterol-lowering medication is bad? HyperTENSION. The name is the problem. Conjures up visions of stress, tension and anxiety, doesn't it? Unfortunately, the term hypertension has confused the public totally. There is a common perception that hypertension is lifestyle and stress-related and nothing that a holiday in the mountains or the seaside wouldn't resolve. Furthermore, in 95% of cases, the disease produces no symptoms. Not for nothing is this condition called the silent killer. It is a major treatable risk factor for stroke, heart attack, heart and kidney failure.

As with high cholesterol, the typical clinical presentation is with a catastrophic event such as death, paralysis, heart attack or unstable angina. Equally disturbing is the recent recognition that high blood pressure doubles your risk of dementia over the age of 65. In 95% of cases we do not know the cause. Blood pressure is controlled by a variety of pressure sensors and chemicals that relay information to the medulla (ignore the word, it isn't particularly necessary to know) of the brain. Located therein is the blood pressure control centre. This regulates blood pressure within a certain range and makes rapid adjustments if stimulated accordingly. All of us will have blood pressure regulated at slightly different baselines. In some individuals the control mechanism regulates pressure at a higher level than others. There is a significant risk of damage to arteries, heart muscle and kidneys with abnormally elevated blood pressure. Blood pressure also rises with age (I am convinced that parenting teenagers is largely responsible, but at this stage, this remains a working hypothesis). The scientific explanation is pretty straightforward. As we age our blood vessels become less elastic and more rigid. As a result they are less able to expand to accommodate the sudden increase in blood volume ejected into them with each heartbeat. Blood pressure rises, particularly during ventricular contraction (known as ventricular systole). Long-term high pressure equals progressive damage to blood vessels.

Five percent of patients have a secondary cause for high blood pressure. Secondary causes include kidney disease, medications (such as the oral contraceptive pill in a small percentage of users, some appetite suppressants, excess alcohol, cocaine, which I admit is not currently widely used for its medicinal properties), unusual forms of adrenal disease, and toxaemia of pregnancy as some examples. These patients can usually be identified by appropriate investigation. The advantage of recognition of these problems is that curative treatment is possible in some cases. What this means is that life-long pill swallowing may not be necessary.

Scenario time again. Sorry, I know this can get painful, but it tends to illustrate the issues clearly. A patient (usually an executive) arrives for his annual company-subsidised medical examination. We chat and joke a bit while I record his medical history. He is a 38 year old new ager. He is a senior vice-president of an advertising company. He jogs 30 miles a week. He is a committed vegetarian. He minimises his salt intake. He meditates for 45 minutes daily. He is arty and creative. His wife steams and boils all his meals. He last ate butter in 1984. His children are compelled to adopt this lifestyle, and eat peanut butter jelly sandwiches and steal cookies whenever they visit friends. I measure his blood pressure. The reading is 162/96. I make a politically correct joke to relax him, chat about the advantages of a high fibre diet for five minutes to relax him, and repeat the measurement. The reading is 167/97. I complete the remainder of the examination. I discuss good things happening in the advertising industry. I measure the blood pressure once again. The reading is166/98. I mention to him that his blood pressure reading seems to be moderately elevated. He is horrified. It must be a consequence of one of a variety of stresses, he says. The cat has gastroenteritis. He is under pressure to attract a big advertising account. The traffic was heavy this morning. His wife is premenstrual. His mother-in-law confessed to him three weeks ago that her daughter should have married better.

I sit down behind the desk and sigh (inaudibly). He is, of course, going to be a nightmare to treat. I explain the essence of hypertension. I use the word high blood pressure so as not to confuse him. He is dumbfounded. He recalls putting sea salt on a parsley pie about three years ago and wonders if that might be the problem. I tell him no. His father had hypertension and died of a stroke at 45. His mother died from a stroke at 70. OK, he admits there are some genetic issues. But he does everything right. And he is an American. He should be entitled to live forever.

We run all the tests. We repeat the blood pressure reading on 17 further occasions. This includes a 24-hr continuous blood pressure recording and a reading while he is meditating with his yoga guru. The blood pressure remains elevated. He discusses the stresses in his life with his therapist, trains even harder, and loses even more weight than necessary. He practically eliminates salt from his diet. He tries herbal therapies by the dozen. After six months he returns for a repeat check-up. The blood pressure is 171/99. His cholesterol is 7mmol/litre. I explain that he has essential hypertension and elevated cholesterol, both of which are inherited. If I am lucky he will consider a trial of drug therapy. Unfortunately, he has moderately severe hypertension and will probably require at least two drugs to control his blood pressure effectively. His other major vascular risk factor, i.e. his high blood cholesterol (in spite of his Bridge on the River Kwai diet) warrants the use of a statin. His risks for an adverse cardiovascular event (particularly a stroke or a heart attack), before the age of 60 certainly justify considering the use of long-term low-dose aspirin therapy. I will clarify the role of aspirin further in a later chapter. As you can imagine it is difficult for any individual who feels at peak mental and physical fitness to be told he requires the life-long consumption of multiple drugs.

OK, let's reiterate. High blood pressure is a silent killer. Blood pressure rises with age, largely because blood vessels become less elastic and stiffer. Reduced elasticity results in a reduced ability of blood vessels to expand to accommodate sudden changes in blood volume created by the pumping action of the heart. At the age of 21 only 1% of the population has high blood pressure. At the age of 60 about 40% of us have high blood pressure. Those of us fortunate enough to live to 80 will have a 60% chance of having high blood pressure. Almost a normal phenomenon of aging, isn't it? Yes, but only if you are happy to die earlier than necessary from a stroke, dementia, a heart attack, heart failure or kidney failure (or all of the above). Remember our ancestors did not recognize the concept of natural death. Death was death, whether it involved an encounter with a sabre-toothed tiger, infection, starvation, cannibalism, murder, or an argument with the mother-in-law. Advanced old age in those days was defined as living beyond the age of 35. The modern long-term disease processes which occur as a consequence of genes, environment, and natural aging, were hardly relevant. In the 19th and early 20th century, myocardial infarction (heart attack) was a very rare cause of death. Now it is our number-one killer.

NO FOLKS this is not only a consequence of lifestyle. It is an age thing. With life expectancies in the 30-40 age range, heart disease barely had a chance. There were too many other competing causes of death in the younger age groups to give it any opportunity. Perhaps this is why we have no genetic memory of the condition and are significantly genetically motivated to eat, eat, and eat. The low cholesterol, high fibre lifestyle hardly provided a survival advantage to our ancestors. Exercise, of course, is still a basic drive and physical fitness undoubtedly improves cardiorespiratory (heart and lung) fitness, muscle and bone strength, and feelings of wellbeing. Those who thrived on activity were almost certainly more likely to be successful hunters and (dare I say it) better lovers. Unfortunately, the competing urges to accumulate and conserve food energy seem to have been even more effective in improving survival and hence the opportunity to pass on the relevant genetic profile.

In the real world the consequences are obvious. A large proportion of patients fail to adhere adequately to therapy. There is a widely held public perception that improving life expectancy requires the development of newer and more effective drugs. This is undoubtedly not the case in the treatment of most cases of hypertension. We have a wide range of effective agents available. They work via widely different mechanisms. Any drug can cause side-effects in a proportion of users but the wide range of modern drugs should practically guarantee safe, convenient (at the very most twice daily), effective therapy. About 40% of patients will require at least two drugs for effective blood pressure control. Doctors know that most patients with hypertension are asymptomatic. It is therefore incumbent upon them to ensure that patients do not suffer side-effects, at the very least for the emotionally intelligent reason that side-effects equal non-adherence to treatment. Naturally, if you don't take the treatment it doesn't work. Important side-effects often overlooked are those that we are kind of embarrassed to shout from our rooftops e.g. impotence. YOU deserve appropriate therapy for life-threatening conditions and you deserve to feel and function normally on such therapy. Even if you don't have medical insurance. And emphasise unacceptable side-effects to your doctor.

Now, why the hell did I say that? Several recent studies have revealed that at least 40% of Americans with health insurance and a diagnosis of hypertension are receiving inadequate therapy. With current state-of-the-art therapy and recent evidence-based (i.e. objective rather than best guess) research, the target for adequate blood pressure control has become lower. In the old days a copout was much easier. Sure, we lowered blood pressure but side-effects such as depression, impotence, breast development in males, increased facial hair in females, and multiple other inflictions were common. This is no longer the case when treatment is prescribed appropriately. Let me spell it out. Target blood pressure should be less than 140/85. In some subgroups such as diabetics with renal disease, 130/80 or less is ideal. And be careful not to take the bumph about stress or doctor-induced (white coat) hypertension too seriously. Labile hypertension (i.e. a normal baseline blood pressure but abnormally high level under emotional stress), also increases the risk of vascular disease. If Brad Pitt knocks your blood pressure through the roof so be it. If a nerd with a white coat and coke bottle glasses does, ensure that at the very least your blood pressure is closely monitored on a regular basis. And consider, at least, non-drug measures of blood pressure control. Or maybe even a pill. (Oh! Oh! I have gone and said the "p" word again).

Non-drug therapy should not be over-emphasised in this book, which is for normal people i.e. those who hate long-term serious self-sacrifice. Of course it has a place, but concerns regarding long-term compliance have been raised, largely because long-term compliance sucks. Anyway for those who prefer the non-drug approach, the following rules apply:

♦ Reduce salt intake to less than 6g a day.

♦ Lose weight through appropriate conventional dieting - see the general guidelines.

♦ Exercise more.

♦ Alcohol: upper limit 30g a day for men and 15g for women (zero for AA members).

♦ Avoid illegal stimulants.

♦ Oral contraceptives and other drugs may be contributing to the problem. Check these out with your doctor. Oral contraceptives are the commonest cause of medication-induced hypertension.

♦ Ignore any ridiculous advice about reducing stress - I mean, how on earth do you measure the relevance of such advice? Any response is unlikely to be of realistic help. In particular, absurd lifestyle changes will turn out to be exactly that - absurd lifestyle changes.

♦ Try not to think of Nicole Kidman or Charlize Theron (if you are a male) and Brad Pitt and Tom Cruise if you are female.

♦ Destroy the picture of your mother-in-law in the hall.

♦ Minimise other risk factors for heart, vascular and kidney disease by reading all the other chapters. This will involve purchasing the book.

The range of available medications includes thiazides, beta-blockers, angiotensin-converting-enzyme (ACE) inhibitors, calcium channel blockers, alpha-adrenergic blockers, vasodilators, angiotensin 2 receptor blockers, centrally acting anti-adrenergics, combined alpha- and beta-blockers, and a range of other older agents. Newer agents are in the pipeline. I have mentioned the different medication types to emphasise the wide range of drugs available to treat hypertension. They work in different ways and have different side-effect profiles. This means that if a particular agent is just not agreeing with you, treatment can be changed to a totally different drug in which the relevant side-effects are unlikely to occur.

These therapies are prescription-based and clearly choice of therapy requires consultation with your M.D. Different drugs are prescribed depending on clinical context. We know, for example, that beta-blockers and ACE inhibitors improve life expectancy following a heart attack even in the absence of pre-existing hypertension, so clearly these would be the preferred agents to use in that particular patient subgroup. Patients with enlarged prostates who wake up to urinate five times a night and have a urinary flow of dribbling proportions would be likely to find that alpha-receptor blockers improve urinary flow rates and lower their blood pressure as well (killing two birds with one stone if you will pardon the expression). I could go on and on about the advantages and disadvantages of the different drug groups but I won't, I promise. Decisions reside with you and your doctor. Before conception, treatment for high blood pressure should be changed to drugs known to be safe during pregnancy.

So:

♦   Have your blood pressure checked and appropriately treated if necessary. A borderline blood pressure requires follow-up. Blood pressure rises with age and therefore annual routine measurement is mandatory. Recognize that hypertension is either not treated or inadequately treated in a large proportion of patients. It is asymptomatic. It is a silent killer (like VAT and credit cards).

Remember folks, heaven can wait.

● Untreated or inadequately treated hypertension is a silent killer.

● Blood pressure levels regarded as acceptable in the past are too high.

● Blood pressure rises with age so 50% of 60 year olds should expect to be on treatment.

● Modern medications save lives and prevent suffering.

● Many people suffering from high blood pressure are not aware of this so routine monitoring is important.

References

1. STAESSEN JA *et al.* Essential Hypertension. *The Lancet* 2003; 361(9369):1629-41.

2. FONAROW GH, HORWICH TB. Prevention of heart failure: effective strategies to combat the growing epidemic. *Rev Cardiovasc Med* 2003; 4(1): 8-17.

3. NEUTEL JM, SMITH DH. Improving patient compliance: a major goal in the management of hypertension. *J Clin Hypertens* 2003; 5(2): 127-32.

4. DOUGLAS JG *et al.* Barriers to blood pressure control in African Americans. Overcoming obstacles is challenging, but target goals can be attained. *Postgrad Med* 2002; 112(4): 51-2, 55, 59-62.

Chapter 8

Aspirin

If aspirin had been discovered ten years ago by the leading lights of the scientific community, it would have been heralded as a great scientific breakthrough. It would have cost a fortune. This drug reduces heart and stroke attack risk in medium and high-risk subgroups. It also improves survival during a heart attack, a thrombotic stroke (stroke caused by a clot rather than a primary bleed into the brain) and unstable angina (a syndrome that often results in heart attack). It has a prophylactic effect in heart attack and stroke survivors. No, this does not mean it acts as a contraceptive in these patients. It reduces their risk of further clinical heart disease and stroke. Great stuff. The drug was in fact discovered over a century ago. It is a modification of salicin, an extract of willow bark. Is that cool or what? A plant extract. This drug is a modified herb and should have endless possibilities as a natural health supplement. The generic name of aspirin is acetylsalicylate. The name aspirin is in fact the first trade name registered to the original manufacturers, Bayer Pharmaceuticals. The drug was of course, used purely as a painkiller until its effect on platelet function was recognized.

I had better elaborate. After all, we doctors have largely lost our aura as the font of all medical wisdom, and you won't take the medication otherwise. Assuming you need it of course. Aspirin in low doses interferes with the tendency of platelets (the small blood cells which play a major role in blood clotting) to stick to one another. In their usual inactivated state, blood platelets do not adhere to one another or the internal lining of blood vessels (known as the vascular endothelium). Any break in the endothelium exposes the underlying tissues to platelets. The platelets bind to the underlying material (in particular a fibre-like material known as collagen) by means of a collagen receptor on the platelet surface. A complex cascade of reactions is then triggered causing platelets to stick to one another and form a "platelet plug". This stabilises further to form a firm clot, effectively plugging the break in the blood vessel wall and hence further bleeding. Now in the normal situation this is a pretty sound idea. Blood carries the nutrients and oxygen (the combustible energy supply, remember) essential for life. The blood vessels are the conduits that convey blood to all the cells of the body. You bleed excessively; you die. Definitely not rocket science. Recently attacked by a Neanderthal, gored by a woolly mammoth, or given birth to quadruplets in 55,000 B.C., you would want a large supply of normally functioning platelets. You really do not want to exsanguinate. You want to survive to the ripe old age of 32 so you can celebrate your twilight years watching your great grandchildren frolic amongst the dung in front of your retirement cave.

But several thousand years on, the world has changed. Neanderthals are extinct. Hardly surprising, is it? Who wants to sleep with a Frankenstein look-alike (even if you are seriously drunk, girls). And woolly mammoths disappeared for different reasons, namely hunting and climate change. But I digress.

Plumbing, antibiotics, etc. have resulted in *Homo sapiens* being a serious long-term survivor. Unfortunately, increasing longevity has a downside. As we age our blood vessels age with us. Hypertension, high blood fats, cigarettes, diabetes, labour-saving devices, inactivity, fast foods, and a range of other issues exacerbate the problem. These multiple conspiracies progressively damage our arterial system. The arteries carry oxygen-containing blood to the body. Fatty (atheromatous) deposits accumulate in artery walls. They weaken the endothelial lining. This results in turbulent flow. Ongoing mechanical stress and possibly inflammation of these fatty plaques aggravates the problem. A crack or rupture in one of these areas activates the platelet/clot mechanism. Arteries at particular risk of this include those supplying the heart and brain.

The consequences of a break in the endothelial (internal) lining of an artery are thus platelet plugging, clot formation and obstruction of the artery. Oh, #%&*! The immediate result is cutting off of the blood supply (and hence oxygen and nutrients) downstream, with ultimate suffocation and death of the supplied area. Clots not uncommonly break up and the restored blood flow will minimise the damage if this occurs while the supplied tissues are still viable.

You happy? Getting to see the bigger picture? A clotting system designed to minimise blood loss in the young and violent is a trifle over-efficient as our arteries age. Given that the risk of violent death in the middle-aged and elderly is markedly less than the risk of fatal heart attack and stroke (except maybe in South Central Los Angeles and parts of the third world), those of us at increased risk of cardiovascular disease need less sticky platelets. A fatty plaque ruptures, less sticky platelets will not adhere to each other in the area of the rupture, which then simply heals. A great clot does not form, the artery does not occlude, and we live to wine, dine and love another day. And that is how aspirin works. It irreversibly acetylates an enzyme called COX (cyclo-oxygenase) 1 and blocks platelet activation. The platelets remain inactive and do not adhere to one another. Paradoxically, it is low doses of aspirin that are effective. Large doses do not work as they modify the endothelial (i.e. inner) lining of arterial walls in such a way that platelets tend to stick to them. The lack of effect of larger doses explains the delayed recognition of aspirin's value in cardiovascular medicine, even though the antiplatelet effect has been recognised for many decades.

So, should we all be popping a third of a regular aspirin a day? No. WHADDAYA MEAN NO! After all this scientific bumph you have forced us to wade through. Like everything in life, there is a downside. Aspirin does increase the risk of peptic ulcer and gastrointestinal haemorrhage. It also marginally increases the risk of primary intracerebral haemorrhage (a stroke from a bleed into the brain tissue rather than a clot in an artery). The individual risk of these side-effects is low and it has been recommended that if your individual risk of heart attack or atherothrombotic stroke (caused by clot and obstruction rather than by bleeding) exceeds 3% in the next five years, you should consider taking prophylactic low-dose aspirin. OK, you clearly should not take aspirin if you are a 16 year old schoolgirl, allergic to aspirin, or a heavyweight boxer. A history of heavy menstrual bleeding, iron deficiency, unexplained anaemia, and an active stomach ulcer would also preclude the use of the drug.

Individuals over the age of 45 with any other risk factor for heart attack or stroke and no contra-indications, should consider taking this drug (after discussion with their doctor). Be clear that this is a recommendation as a primary preventive measure in individuals with no known pre-existing cardiovascular disease. Patients with known cardiovascular disease should be on the drug for secondary prevention as a routine, unless clear contra-indications exist. LOW doses work. Do not exceed 150mg per day (half a standard aspirin). Because side-effects of bleeding increase with increasing dose, I advise my patients to take 75mg to 100mg per day. These tiny doses have been quaintly remarketed at hugely inflated prices as cardio-protective agents. An option is to purchase 300mg aspirin tablets in bulk at your local supermarket and take approximately one third of a tablet a day.

Are there any other benefits of this new wonder drug? Well there is some evidence (suggestive but not conclusively proven) that low-dose aspirin also reduces the risk of bowel cancer slightly. A recent study also suggested a reduction in the risk of cancer of the throat and oesophagus (gullet) in long-term low-dose aspirin users. Not bad for a modified extract of willow bark. Even the alternative care practitioners and homeopaths should be impressed.

● If you are at increased risk for heart or vascular disease there needs to be a very good reason why you are not taking low-dose aspirin.

References

1.   HENNEKENS CH. Update on aspirin in the treatment and prevention of cardiovascular disease. *Am J Manag Care* 2002; 8(22 Suppl): S691-700.
2.   WEISMAN SM, GRAHAM DY. Evaluation of the benefits and risks of low-dose aspirin in the secondary prevention of cardiovascular and cerebrovascular events. *Arch Int Med* 2002; 162(19): 2197-202.

Chapter 9

Can I offer you a light?

Oh! Oh! This chapter could get painful. Look, folks I'm a M.D. I can hardly avoid including a chapter on the pleasures and perils of smoking. Unless of course, the tobacco corporations offer to buy me out. That would only be a realistic option if the book became a million seller.

Anyway, where were we? Ah, yes - tobacco. Modern western society is very, very, very against the idea of cigarette smoking. The more politically correct the nation (or individual), the greater the ire directed against smokers. And it isn't going to get better. Serial killer? Poor bloke must have some deep psychological angst as a consequence of childhood abuse or trauma, even if he also lights fires and drowns kittens. But a smoker has no excuse. She is a dirty, smelly, tobacco-stained degenerate who poisons our air. She partakes in the most disgusting habit imaginable. She is not welcome in our homes and offices. She is never pitied. She lacks self-discipline. Imagine Mother Theresa as a woman with a weakness for cheap cigarillos. The accolades would have dried up. Quickly. Society should not have to tolerate such people. Even the sight of a smoker nipping out of the office to stand on the street at -5°C isn't enough. Bring back stoning - to the Western world I mean.

Yet Hitler was abstemious. Churchill was a smoker. Take that, PC brigade. You will never know the pleasures of a relaxing post-coital puff, or coffee with that first cigarette after a long, exhausting working day.

Why don't we start with the good news about smoking? It is a very effective form of taxation. It reduces long-term pension payouts because smokers die younger (after paying all that tax on cigarettes) and so don't clog up retirement hospitals and such-like. It appears to reduce the risk of acquiring Parkinson's disease, ulcerative colitis (a type of inflammatory bowel disease), an unusual condition called extrinsic allergic alveolitis, and possibly Alzheimer's disease (poor evidence base with lots of potentially confounding issues, e.g. if you die at 55 from lung cancer, you are less likely to live to an age where Alzheimer's disease manifests). Also of course, it is enjoyable. Addictive, yes, and bad for you, yes, but enjoyable.

The downside of smoking is large. Apart from the growing and increasingly self-righteous crusade against smokers, there are many ways in which smoking can kill you. It probably reduces average life expectancy by seven years. It increases the risk of being seriously ill during most of your retirement (if you get there). We should all know the two essentials of a happy retirement, namely health and wealth. Disabling lung and cardiac conditions limit the fun of retiring to a condo in Florida, playing bridge and golf during the day and having outrageous sex with your 84 year old husband at night. It increases the risk of heart attack, stroke and a range of cancers too long to list, but in particular lung cancer (the mother of all cancers), cancers of the mouth, the throat, the bladder, the oesophagus etc. And it progressively corrodes your bronchial tubes and lung tissues to cause chronic bronchitis and emphysema. As a result, your ability to exercise and swing from the chandelier is substantially curtailed. This progresses over time to reduced tolerance of any exertion (such as getting to the post box or the toilet). Next comes shortness of breath at rest and then, ultimately, suffocation. Small fine-boned women who smoke seem particularly at risk of emphysema. Oh, and by the way, screening programs to detect lung cancer early are not effective. Lung cancer remains the commonest overall cause of cancer-related deaths. This cancer kills more people than breast cancer, prostate cancer and bowel cancer combined, simply because of its aggressive nature and high mortality. And not even the recently retired Iraqi Minister of Information would be able to convince us otherwise. The facts speak for themselves.

There are significant financial implications of smoking for decades. Tobacco is taxed like nothing else in OECD countries and smoking has become a very expensive habit. Given the time value of money, regular monthly investing of money that would otherwise have been spent on cigarettes probably totals half a million US dollars for a pack-a-day smoker.

Hey, what is this, a horror story? Do you think I haven't tried to quit? It's just that cigarettes are so damned addictive. Really, Doc. The truth is that there is no totally painless way to stop smoking. Let's talk through the issues related to stopping an addiction. It's here. In the book. A bit like the small print in an insurance contract. And like the small print in the insurance contract, you ignore it at your peril.

Cigarettes are incredibly addictive. Studies on rats confirm that it is easier to quit cocaine than cigarettes. When confronting addictions, there are several phases that the addict (or whatever) tends to move through, during the withdrawal process. Firstly, there is the phase of pre-contemplation. During this phase the individual has not even contemplated quitting. She is happy and enjoying the delights of the substance. Given the adverse publicity and attitudes regarding smoking, you would need to be either a Martian or on death row, not to be aware of current public perceptions regarding smokers. The next phase is contemplation. You are starting to feel like hell in the mornings. Your non-smoking partner is bitching non-stop about the habit. All those dating agencies demand non-smoking, six foot four athletic geniuses, who enjoy dancing, dining out, long walks along lonely beaches at sunset or quiet nights at home. Preferably in the millionaire bracket. The required female equivalent would make Brittney Spears look frumpy. Yeah, we've all seen the ads. Anyway, amazingly enough, on your first date through the agency (you have lied about the smoking, of course) you get the partner from heaven. You are suddenly in love. So you take multiple toilet breaks to sneak a quick one and chew peppermints before returning to the table. By this time your date from heaven assumes you have a prostate problem (if you are male), stress urinary incontinence (if you are female), or that you have a serious cocaine habit. Nevertheless, because of your stunning good looks and sparkling personality, the wonder date agrees to a second meeting (thinking there is an excellent chance of getting a lot more physically intimate if you are female, or that you are very, very rich, if you are male). So you need to quit. Next step in the process is setting a quit date. A bad time to contemplate quitting is just before Xmas and the holiday period. Similarly, don't try to quit just after a job loss, at the time of your first AA meeting, during a divorce or any other particularly stressful period in your life, or during the recovery phase from depression or any other significant psychiatric illness. You need to be emotionally ready. Set a quit date when you are in the zone physically, mentally and emotionally.

Is there a withdrawal syndrome? Of course. Your body has adapted to the expectation of a regular nicotine supply. All those little chemical transmitters and receptors that regulate mood, emotion, concentration, sleep patterns and energy levels are expecting a nicotine hit 10-20 times a day. The classic withdrawal symptoms include daytime fatigue, insomnia, irritability, depressive symptoms and difficulty in concentrating. They can persist for weeks or months and are unpleasant. In fact they can be excruciating. Without chemical support, successful quit rates are about 5% per year. Not good. But us cunning nerds (i.e. doctors) have devised strategies to improve success rates. You need nicotine supplements in gradually decreasing doses over a period of several months. Modes of delivery include absorption via skin patches, nicotine puffers, and chewing gum. Additional drug therapy is necessary to boost quit rates. Medications that have been shown to be effective include the antidepressants bupropion and nortriptyline. Both are prescription medications. Unless there are clear medical contra-indications, use all available resources. And hang in there. Brief relapses are common. Success rates with medical supplementation are in the region of 25-30% at one year.

That's the bottom line, folks. It is tough. The choices are yours. And remember, smoking is not a moral issue. Ignore the PC brigade. The issues are health-related. Be courteous, however, when with non-smokers. There is a small but significant increase in absolute risk for some smoking-related illnesses in passive smokers. Sneak outside for a drag.

OK, enough of the small print. I am starting to feel sanctimonious and this is undoubtedly one of the most undesirable traits in a doctor.

P.S. Did someone mention weight gain during quitting? I thought I might skip that part as it is a disincentive to stop, but being a doctor and also deeply moral, I had better tell you about it. Smokers are on average, several kilograms lighter than non-smokers. Nicotine increases the body's metabolic rate, so calories are burned up more rapidly. The munchies can be a problem during quitting too. As a result, most people will gain 2-3kg on stopping smoking. Unfortunately, a small minority (about 10%) gains considerably more. Body weight needs to be closely monitored during quitting. Most women do not want to look like enormous beach balls so substantial weight gain can be seriously counter-productive, and strongly predicts failure to quit. If significant weight gain occurs, use all my tricks listed in the dietary section. Cosmetically it isn't all one-way traffic though. Decades of smoking cause the tired wrinkled facial features described in the medical literature as smoker's face. Long-term smokers invariably look older than they are. Think back to a movie star who retained the appearance of youthful beauty at 50 and who was also a heavy smoker. I can't recall any. And that's in spite of all the options of modern plastic surgery.

- Cigarette smoking reduces life expectancy by about seven years and often destroys quality of life for many years prior to that.
- Quitting is hard but with support and appropriate drug therapy is achievable.
- Nicotine replacement therapy combined with other drug therapy definitely improves quit rates.

References

1. AIZEN E, GILHAR A. Smoking effect on skin wrinkling in the aged population. *Int J Dermatol* 2001; 40(7): 431-3.
2. BRAUNWALD E *et al. Principles of Internal Medicine*, 15th ed. McGraw-Hill, New York, 2001.
3. PRICE D, DUERDEN M. Chronic obstructive pulmonary disease. *BMJ* 2003; 326(7398): 1046-7.
4. CORNUZ J *et al.* Cost-effectiveness analysis of the first-line therapies for nicotine dependence. *Eur J Clin Pharmcol* 2003; May 21 [Epub ahead of print].

Chapter 10

Whaddya mean you forgot to take a drink last night?

Finally, something easy. Alcohol. The nectar of the gods. A drug with a wide range of tasty formulations, unequivocal health benefits in well-defined patient populations, and that doesn't need a prescription. Price can be a problem, depending on the formulation of choice, but most individuals are prepared to go to significant lengths to adhere to this therapy. Regrettably, a small proportion of users (actually about 10%) becomes a trifle overexuberant in partaking of this wonder drug and develop problems pertaining to addiction or abuse. Like any drug, alcohol isn't a treatment for everyone. OK, I admit I am being a bit of a party-pooper but if you were aware that I am currently wearing a nicotine patch, you might be a trifle more tolerant.

Adults who drink mild to moderate amounts of alcohol on a regular basis, live, on average, about three years longer than teetotallers. When this was demonstrated, the results were treated with considerable circumspection, particularly by the Women's Temperance League and the Salvation Army. The Irish however, celebrated the good news with their usual enthusiasm. Most protestants, on the other hand, find it hard to believe that things that we enjoy can be good for us. I suppose John Calvin must take some of the blame for this. Further research was undertaken and subjected to detailed analysis to ensure that confounding factors were not the cause of the findings. We have all heard Disraeli's quote: "There are lies, damned lies, and statistics." There were several possible confounding factors. The first possibility is that many of the teetotallers were ex-alcoholics with significant underlying medical illness as a consequence. Such individuals would be expected to have a reduced life expectancy and thus skew the results to produce an outcome favouring the alcohol consumer group. This was found not to be the case. The second possibility is that most teetotallers in the western world are rigid, inflexible and self-righteous individuals, prone to personality traits including perfectionism, anxiety and depression. Personality type is extremely difficult to measure quantitatively and precisely in a scientific way, so valid studies are difficult to undertake. We do know that individuals prone to depressive illness have a reduced life expectancy, even if suicide is excluded from the equation. We also know that patients who develop depression following myocardial infarction have a reduced life expectancy unexplained by other factors. However, even in societies where alcohol consumption is low in the general population, regular mild to moderate consumption appears to confer a survival advantage.

If an agent appears to confer a survival advantage, it is reassuring to at least have a working hypothesis as to why this might be so. Low doses of alcohol increase HDL cholesterol levels. Remember HDL cholesterol? Yeah, the good guy. High levels are inversely associated with the risk of heart attack and stroke. Presumably this is the major mechanism by which alcohol confers a survival advantage. Other possible mechanisms include changes in clotting mechanisms. Whoopee! Crack open the Moet! Knock back a Bud or two! Let's have a party! If God wanted us all to have blood fat abnormalities, he wouldn't have invented alcohol.

Now for the detailed advice and the risks. The widespread use of alcohol in society is a mixed blessing, as noted in the first paragraph. Ninety percent of the drinking population have no problem with consumption. They use alcohol as a social lubricant and a relaxant. It helps them unwind. They have a couple of drinks and feel good. They stop. It's easy. You offer them another drink and they say no. These individuals are mild to moderate consumers of alcohol. Mild to moderate consumption of alcohol means a maximum of 30g a day on average for males, and 10-15g a day on average for females. This translates into two and a half beers, glasses of wine or Whiskies for men and one glass of wine for women. Consumption on any single occasion should not exceed four standard drinks. Let's face it, for the above group that's plenty. No problemo. If you fall into this group in terms of your drinking style and have some risk of cardiovascular disease, this is the prescription for you. If you have absolutely no risk of heart disease or stroke (for example, if you are a 14 year old schoolgirl) this clearly doesn't apply. So don't even ask.

10 Whaddya mean you forgot to take a drink last night?

Ten percent of us actually can't control the booze. We have a genetic predisposition to alcoholism. This is under-recognized because most alcoholics are not skid row specials. They are often highly successful people. Ninety-seven percent are employed. They often don't drink during the day (until lunch at least.) They finish work and pop off to the local for eight Margheritas, or home for 20 beers. They pass out at 11p.m. They feel like hell in the morning but get up and go to work.

Their ability to hold their drink is unbelievable. They don't have a couple of Scotches and feel tipsy. In fact they feel like another couple of Scotches. And then another couple. After twelve Scotches they feel like the little Jewish lady does after a thimble of sherry. Merry, and perhaps a bit silly. After 16 drinks they get a bit slurry. And perhaps cantankerous. But they can't turn down the next drink. And so it goes. The illness is progressive and has multiple implications socially, matrimonially, economically, possibly criminally, and of course, healthwise. For these poor devils, one drink is too many and a thousand is never enough. Abstinence is the ideal management for alcoholism. But it is hard. Relapses or slips (mini-relapses) are common. The condition is a chronic illness and needs to be recognised as such. Alcoholics who continue to drink have an average reduction in life expectancy of 15 years. The leading causes of death include heart disease, cancer, accidents, suicide, liver cirrhosis (liver failure) and inflammation of the pancreas. The vast majority of alcoholics are heavy cigarette smokers, which undoubtedly explains some of the association with heart disease and cancer. After all, I have just explained that mild to moderate alcohol consumption reduces the risk of heart attack and stroke. However, heavy sustained alcohol use can cause hypertension and damage heart muscle. Similarly, heavy alcohol consumption increases the risk of some cancers, such as cancer of the liver.

OK, folks that's the story. Aged over 40, no personal history of problems with alcohol and no private or religious issues relating to alcohol, take the medication. In the evenings preferably. With a bit of background jazz.

Does the formulation matter? There have been suggestions that wine is more effective than beer or spirits, possibly due to the fact that wine contains anti-oxidants. The evidence is not compelling however, and should not influence your choice.

If you have been unfortunate enough to have serious problems with alcohol, then this clearly isn't an option for you. Use AA or other support groups to help you. We have other options to help you to live long and enriching lives. And as the Irish would say, I am sorry for your troubles.

● Moderate alcohol consumption improves life expectancy by several years by reducing the risk of heart and vascular disease.

References

1.   DUGGIRALA K *et al*. Alcohol and coronary artery disease. *N Engl J Med* 2003 348(17): 1719-22; author reply 1719-22.
2.   JACKSON VA *et al*. Alcohol consumption and mortality in men with preexisting cerebrovascular disease. *Arch Intern Med* 2003;163(10): 1189-93.
3.   VOGEL RA. Alcohol, heart disease, and mortality: a review. *Rev Cardiovasc Med* 2002; 3(1): 7-13.

Chapter 11

Diabetes mellitus

This is a short chapter. The aim in life is to avoid diabetes mellitus, if at all possible. There is however, a substantial genetic predisposition to Type II diabetes mellitus, in particular. The risk is inherited as part of the metabolic syndrome genetic package in most cases. If a parent or sibling has Type II diabetes, the risk of the disease developing in a particular individual is about 45%. We have talked about diet in earlier chapters. Definitely not painless, but do your best. Can you avoid Type II diabetes if genetically predisposed? Yes, or at least delay it. The incidence of Type II diabetes in Europe following the food rationing in World War II was about a third of that prior to the war. Weight gain is undoubtedly a major risk factor. Oh great, I hear you thinking. He promises us a way to avoid diabetes and now he wants us to declare war on Germany. As we have discussed, long-term successful adherence to a slimming diet is extremely challenging for the average human (and by definition almost all of us are average) with very high failure rates. It clearly can't be the only focus. And this is why diabetic patients have been so disadvantaged in the past. Doctors did not think laterally and were not aggressive in the management of other risk factors contributing to diabetic complications. It was all diet and sugar levels.

Fortunately, that is changing, but it behoves diabetics to be aware of all aspects of management of their condition and to expect best care, even if it becomes necessary to demand it. All diabetics need a doctor expert in the management of the condition to be involved in their care. A team approach is best and includes, in addition, nurse diabetic practitioners, dieticians, family physicians, podiatrists, ophthalmologists etc. The most important member of that team is you. There is class I evidence emphasising that involving the patient in all aspects of disease management improves outcomes. Understand your disease and ensure that you participate in all management decisions.

Type II diabetes mellitus develops over years, from a state of healthy blood sugar control, to impaired control, followed by full-blown diabetes mellitus. Type II diabetes is diagnosed, on average, about nine years after illness onset. For this reason some individuals already have complications of the condition at the time of diagnosis. The disease tends to be progressive. This means that dietary control may be satisfactory in the first instance, but as the disease progresses, oral medications and/or insulin injection therapy may become necessary to achieve satisfactory blood sugar control.

How does Type II diabetes kill? Heart attack and stroke are the most common causes of death. Poor circulation involving the feet and kidney failure are less common causes. There is now unequivocal evidence that all adult diabetic patients should be on a range of medications, apart from those necessary to control blood sugar. I will not expand on blood sugar control and the range of treatments for this further, as these are beyond the scope of this book and will be the co-responsibility of the diabetic team and the patient.

Now, for the painless part - medications that are easy to take and which should make diabetics live longer, if simply swallowed once a day (assuming of course the individual has no contra-indications to such treatment).

The list includes:

♦ An ACE (angiotensin-converting-enzyme) inhibitor or an angiotensin 2 receptor blocker. These prevent progressive kidney damage and should be used even if blood pressure is normal.

♦ Low-dose aspirin - for reasons alluded to earlier in the book.

♦ A HMG CoA reductase inhibitor i.e. a statin to lower blood cholesterol (even if your blood fats are in the so-called normal range).

♦ Target blood pressure should be less than 130/80. Unacceptably high blood pressures have been regarded as acceptable in the past.

Diabetics need all the options available and perfect blood pressure control is obligatory.

♦ For patients with raised fasting blood sugar or impaired glucose tolerance (let's call these an indication of impending diabetes mellitus), a drug called metformin should be considered. There is some evidence that this may delay progression to overt diabetes mellitus. Newer drugs with the same potential benefits are currently undergoing research.

♦ Don't forget the Scotch in moderation, but count the calories contained therein.

● All diabetics should be taking low-dose aspirin, a statin, an ACE inhibitor and moderate amounts of alcohol, unless there are compelling reasons not to do so.

References

1. SOLOMON CG. Editorial: Reducing Cardiovascular risk in Type 2 Diabetes. *NEJM* 2003; 348(5): 457-9.
2. RACHMANI R *et al.* Teaching patients to monitor their risk factors retards the progression of vascular complications in high-risk patients with Type 2 diabetes mellitus. *Diabet Med* 2002; 19: 385-92.

Chapter 12

Other issues related to cardiovascular risk

Homocysteine! Never heard of it prior to reading this book, I bet? Well, let me tell you that there seems to be a relationship between high plasma homocysteine levels and atherosclerosis - potentially leading to a heart attack or stroke. It is unclear if the relationship is incidental or causal. Nevertheless, we know that rare hereditary conditions in which homocysteine levels are extremely high are associated with a markedly increased risk for heart attack and stroke. Homocysteine seems to increase the risk of damaging arterial walls and also the risk of arterial thrombosis (blood clotting). Homocysteine is an amino acid that is necessary for the synthesis of cysteine, another building block essential for life. Diseases that cause markedly elevated homocysteine levels are rare, as mentioned above. Nevertheless, more subtle variations in the way our bodies process this agent can lead to a moderately increased level of homocysteine in the blood, with increase in vascular risk.

You will appreciate, I hope, that my typing speed is ten words a minute and I would not be telling you all this if there was no opportunity for treating moderate elevations in plasma homocysteine. Levels can be reduced by folate and vitamin B6 and B12 supplementation. Yes, I am recommending vitamin supplementation. A nice natural supplement. See chapter 3 for further details regarding vitamin supplementation in general.

Lipoprotein (a) is a minor lipoprotein. High levels are associated with an increase in risk of atherosclerosis. The mechanism is unclear but may be related to the fact that lipoprotein (a) interferes with clot breakdown. Routine screening is not recommended because no treatment is available. I believe that approach is short-sighted. If I had an elevated lipoprotein (a), was over 40, or had any other risk factor for heart attack or stroke, I would take low-dose aspirin, and any other necessary treatment to minimise my individual risk.

There is ongoing investigation into the causes of atherosclerosis and there are a number of theoretical associations for which there is no definite proof currently. These include infection or low-grade inflammation of fatty plaques, and unusual blood chemical abnormalities that predispose to clotting. There are also natural risk factors that we cannot avoid. These include aging (no, Botox doesn't help), gender (being male), and some genetic factors. So let's ignore these. There were great hopes that hormone replacement therapy would be effective in preventing cardiovascular disease in post-menopausal women, but, sadly, recent evidence refutes this.

Emotional stress is often ascribed as a cause of heart disease. The difficulties in scientifically evaluating the impact of stress are multiple. First of all, how the hell do we define stress? Some individuals thrive on pressure whereas others disintegrate. Responses to different challenges vary, even in the same individual. A mathematics boffin might experience no negative emotions at the thought of an algebra examination but develop a panic attack during a public speech. For most politicians the reverse would no doubt be true. Studies to define the issue further have compared the two basic personality types, namely type A and type B personality. Type A personalities are competitive, go-getter, ambitious individuals, driven by a sense of time urgency and displaying the rather unfortunate tendency to free-floating hostility. Type B personalities are laid-back, sluggish, relaxed and lacking in drive and ambition. Attempts to correlate personality type with cardiac risk have been confounded by the complexities of defining personality and methodological limitations.

It appears that acute stress does not cause atherosclerosis to develop. How many 22 year olds have a heart attack before a university examination? Nevertheless, if you have the disease and really lose your cool, the sudden rise in blood pressure and consequent vascular turbulence can cause a fatty (i.e. atherosclerotic) plaque to crack, with subsequent blood clot formation and a full blown heart attack. So do we advise people to avoid stress after a heart attack? Actually, not usually in the medium to long-term. Simply because when we do, we are basically talking crap. Imagine telling the type A personality who derives her stimulation, social kudos, and six-figure income from her job, to sell up and head for a condo on the coast. The stress would kill her. In addition, beta-blocker drugs, in particular, are extremely effective in protecting the heart and arterial system from the effects of stress. Studies following heart attack survivors have shown no survival advantage whatsoever for type B personalities. By using appropriate preventive medication you shouldn't be at significant risk of atherosclerosis anyway (well, at least not until you are senile).

So you want to know more about stress. We are all familiar with the typical symptoms of stress. They are the consequence of increased adrenalin secretion and are the body's response mechanism to prepare for fight or flight in response to a perceived threat. The symptoms include feelings of fear, being on edge, jumpy and nervous, as well as physical sensations such as "butterflies" in the pit of the stomach, muscle tension, tremulousness and palpitations. If inappropriate, exaggerated or prolonged, they can certainly become distressing. As a general rule of thumb, stress (anxiety in medical parlance) becomes a disability if it interferes with either your quality of life or your ability to function effectively. Specific (and sensible) therapy for the stress should then be considered. This discussion leads very effectively into the next chapter, where the effects of a far more sinister emotion are discussed.

- Have your homocysteine and lipoprotein (a) levels checked.
- Vitamin B and folate supplements are helpful for elevated homocysteine levels.
- Consider low-dose aspirin if lipoprotein (a) levels are elevated.
- Do not adopt ridiculous and unsubstantiated advice about avoiding stress.

References

1. HAYNES WG. Hyperhomocysteinemia, vascular function and atherosclerosis: effects of vitamins. *Cardiovasc Drugs Ther* 2002;16(5): 391-9.
2. YEH ET, PALUSINSKI RP. C-reactive protein: the pawn has been promoted to queen. *Curr Atheroscler Rep* 2003; 5(2): 101-5.

Chapter 13

Depression - fighting the black suffocation

Depression. Such a tragically misunderstood, underdiagnosed and stigmatising condition. The name is part of the problem, similar to the misleading name for high blood pressure i.e. hypertension. For goodness sake, can't you just pull yourself together? We all get miserable at times. So snap out of it. And don't use that word. Everyone will think the whole family is crazy. Or worse, your mother will blame me. After all I've done for .... blah, blah, blah.

Why the hell am I mentioning depression? I thought we were focusing on physical illness. Not people with issues. It's simple, really. Depression is unequivocally an illness, produces long-term suffering in many of those afflicted, destroys careers, relationships and lives, and is a major player as one of the most prevalent diseases of the new millennium. More importantly, because it is usually recurrent, it can predispose the victim to years of unnecessary suffering.

When evaluating the impact of an illness, we try to measure its effect not only in terms of life expectancy, but also on quality of life. The acronym QALY is now common medical parlance. This stands for quality adjusted life years. As mentioned previously, these are the good years when life is really worth living. Depression causes a greater loss of QALYs than almost any other illness. About 15-20% of the population will experience an episode of major depression during their lives. The condition is more common in women. There are a variety of types of depressive illness. I plan to focus on unipolar major depression and dysthymia (low grade chronic depression) in this book, because these conditions are the most prevalent in the community, are frequently overlooked, inadequately treated, and, if identified, can transform and save lives. So what did you expect, a laugh a minute in a chapter on depressive illness? If you are Ms. (or Mr.) Happy and live on the sunny side of the street, be my guest and skip the chapter

The causes of depression are not well understood but it is clear that both nature and nurture play a role in predisposing to the illness. The disease is commoner in identical twins (about a 50% chance that if one twin has the illness, the other will develop it) than non-identical twins (the chance of both non-identical twins developing the illness is about 20%). Individuals in the same family may be exposed to similar environmental influences, and, in order to isolate the effects of genetic inheritance, studies of twins adopted into different family environments have been undertaken. Thus each individual twin grows up in a different environment. Furthermore, because identical twins are genetically identical, whereas non-identical twins obviously share less genetic characteristics, a strong genetic influence on the cause of depression would be reflected in differing prevalence of the illness between the two twin groups. As mentioned above, study results have consistently demonstrated a 50% chance of developing the disease in adopted identical twins and a 20% chance in adopted non-identical twins. These results clearly confirm that genes play a role in predisposition to depression. Precisely how they do is unclear. A wide range of chemical messengers and receptors for these messengers exist in the brain. There are many different types and groupings of nerve cells, extensive and interlinking nerve networks, and multiple chemicals and nerves outside the brain that can impact on brain functioning. So it isn't easy to sort out the issues, and a considerable amount of further research is necessary to clarify the multiple mechanisms involved in causing depression. Two chemicals in particular, namely serotonin and noradrenaline (norepinephrine), seem to be implicated in regulation of mood, and low levels of both, but serotonin in particular, correlate well with depressive symptoms. Most currently available antidepressants increase the levels of one or both of these agents in areas of the brain associated with regulation of emotion (the limbic system, raphe nuclei, superior central nucleus, neocortex and entorhinal cortex - see, you shouldn't have asked).

So what the hell does all that infer? Basically anyone can develop a depressive illness given sufficient stress, but the threshold varies considerably. Some people appear genetically predisposed to developing depression at much lower stress levels than others. Are there any stressors particularly likely to trigger an episode of depression in a vulnerable individual? There has been considerable research in this area and the evidence is not absolute. Nevertheless, you have to be pretty stupid to believe negative life events do not increase the risk of depression. This applies particularly to the first episode of illness. Your dog dies, your husband leaves you for a 20 year old blond with an IQ of 18 and all the other attributes that middle-aged men find so attractive, you lose your job and your parents die. You develop a lump in your breast. All in the same month.

And some 26 year old scientist with the emotional quotient of a dead fish wonders if the primary problem is low serotonin levels. Stressors most likely to be associated with increased risk of depression in adults include:

♦ Parental loss before adolescence.

♦ A deprived, unstable childhood home environment.

♦ Major negative life events such as bereavement, job loss, loss of social status, marital stress, separation, divorce, emigration and social isolation.

How is depression identified? In the past it was easy for doctors to diagnose depression. We guessed. We missed most of the cases that way and treated other individuals inappropriately. The diagnosis currently requires the satisfying of certain criteria. These have been well validated and are sensitive and specific for the diagnosis. Use of quality criteria means that missing or mislabelling of patients should be rare. Unfortunately, depression remains seriously under-diagnosed and under-treated. The DSM 4 criteria of the American Psychiatric Association * are widely used for the diagnosis of depressive illness. I have simplified the medical terminology and provided examples to promote easier comprehension of the jargon.

The criteria to confirm the diagnosis of a major depressive episode are as follows:

Five (or more) of the following symptoms should have been present during the same two-week period and represent a change from previous functioning; at least one of the symptoms should be either depressed mood or loss of pleasure (known as anhedonia).

Each symptom should be present most days and for much of the day.

♦ Depressed mood or anhedonia.

♦ Loss of interest or pleasure in all, or almost all, activities. An example would be of a fanatical sports fan who can no longer feel any pleasure at his teams' successes. Libido also takes a nosedive.

♦ Unexplained weight loss when not dieting and/or loss of appetite, or unexplained increase in appetite or unexplained weight gain. Craving carbohydrates is not uncommon in the latter group. Weight change should be at least 5% from baseline bodyweight to be significant.

♦ Insomnia (inability to sleep) or hypersomnia (excessive sleepiness). Some people have a combination of the two. They want to sleep all the time, but, when they get to bed, find they can't. Early morning waking (terminal insomnia) is also common.

♦ Psychomotor agitation (a distressing feeling of anxiety and restlessness) or psychomotor retardation (a feeling of being mentally and physically slowed down).

♦ Loss of energy and fatigue. Wake up tired, go to bed tired, always tired. Even a good night's sleep will not alleviate the fatigue.

♦ Feelings of low self-esteem (feeling absolutely worthless) and excessive or inappropriate guilt for real or perceived failings.

♦ Diminished ability to think or concentrate, with forgetfulness and indecisiveness. This is observable by others and not only the patient.

♦ Recurrent thoughts of death, thoughts of suicide with or without a formal plan, or actual suicide attempt.

Diagnostic criteria for dysthymia (ongoing low grade depression) include the following:

Depressed mood for most of the day, for more days than not, as indicated by subjective account or observation by others, for at least two years. In children and adolescents, the mood can be irritable and duration should be at least one year.

Presence, while depressed, of at least two of the following:

♦ Poor appetite or overeating.

♦ Insomnia or hypersomnia.

♦ Low energy or fatigue.

♦ Low self-esteem.

♦ Poor concentration or indecisiveness.

♦ Feelings of hopelessness.

During the period of the illness the person has never been without the symptoms for more than two months at a time.

The most important diagnostic criteria for a serious major depression, and the most devastating of the symptoms, are anhedonia (as mentioned above, the inability to experience any pleasure and, yes, that includes winning the Lotto), total loss of all self-esteem, and profoundly depressed mood. This is useful in the distinction between depression and bereavement. Your dog dies, you feel sad. The sadness is not associated with feelings of worthlessness, hopelessness and anhedonia. You win the Lotto or have a good meal a few days later; you are capable of deriving pleasure from the event. This distinction is crucial. Imagine feeling that you will never again be able to derive pleasure or joy from anything. And that you are worthless. And useless. And that continuing to live in this desperate scenario is pointless and unendurable. Hardly surprising that the lifetime suicide rate for patients afflicted by depressive illness is 15%.

If you have dysthymia, you are likely to be perceived as a miserable #%&*, a generally unlikeable, irritable, unhappy piece of work, forever moaning and groaning and seldom satisfied. However, you do have some mood reactivity. If you win the Lotto you feel good. For a week or two. Then life reverts back to the status quo. The default mood is one of low-grade sadness. Are you just a pessimist for whom the glass is always half empty? Possibly. If you do satisfy the criteria for dysthymia, however, you perhaps have a condition for which treatment that will improve the quality of your life is available.

If depressive illness is so disabling why the hell did it not disappear as a result of the process of natural selection? After all, living with someone who is depressed sucks. It drags you down. Who wouldn't prefer Mr. Happy next door? I can only presume that negativistic thinking has been of some advantage in perpetuating the trait. Take for example, Noah (of the Ark fame). While the rest of the world was living it up in glorious sunshine, Noah took a dim view of the future. He did not overindulge or celebrate life. Worse case scenario was his initial response to any new challenge. So he built an Ark instead and survived. The pessimistic view is often more realistic than a rampantly optimistic point of view. This is particularly important when choosing a stockbroker. If you learn nothing else from this book, remember this: never, never, never choose an optimistic stockbroker. But I digress. A pessimistic outlook is appropriate in certain scenarios. It becomes inappropriate where it is excessive, inaccurate, enduring and all pervasive. Absolute loss of ability to enjoy anything and feelings of utter worthlessness are the cornerstone of depressive illness. This interferes with ability to function and life appreciation. As the illness evolves it develops a life of its own, distorting perceptions and concepts of self and reality. Instead of a chilly breeze, it becomes a force ten arctic gale at midnight, tearing away the fabric of self and soul.

Depressive illness is not a one-off disease. It is not comparable to, say, pneumonia, where you get sick, we give you an antibiotic and you recover fully. A typical pneumonia is a single episode of illness that does not confer any increase in risk of recurrence in the future. The disease model of depression is now thought to resemble chronic conditions such as diabetes and rheumatoid arthritis, rather than pneumonia. It is chronic and recurrent. After a single episode of depression, the risk for a second episode increases substantially. Two episodes increase the risk further. The initial episode appears to be more likely to be precipitated by a life crisis, whereas further episodes less commonly have a clearly defined triggering stressor. It is not clear why this is the case but it is thought that the multitude of hormonal, nerve cell, and chemical changes that occur during the illness can change brain functioning permanently. As a result, the emotional default setting of the brain might be geared towards depression. Recognising this has been critical in changing the approach to managing the condition.

What are the wider implications of this illness?

♦ Fifteen percent of individuals with a lifetime history of depression die from suicide.

♦ Even if suicide is excluded, life expectancy of patients with depression is three years less than average. The reasons are not clear but may be related to toxic effects of some of the older antidepressant drugs on the heart, the effects of stress in increasing the risk of heart disease, and the possibility that depression suppresses immunity. Patients who develop depression after a heart attack have a reduced life expectancy.

♦ Drug abuse: self medicating with a strong Bourbon, a snort of coke or a joint, simply to feel OK can evolve into a life-threatening habit. Depression increases the lifetime risk of substance abuse to 50%.

♦ QALYs. Depression takes great chunks out of an individual's quality of life. It can destroy self-esteem, career prospects, marriages, parenting relationships etc.

How do we manage this illness?

The median age of the first episode of unipolar major depression is about 40 but can occur anytime. Untreated, most patients will eventually recover after about nine months. Effective antidepressant therapy can shorten the duration of the acute illness to six weeks. It is important that treatment is continued for 6-12 months. A shorter duration of therapy is almost always followed by relapse. Given the high incidence of recurrence, prophylactic therapy should be discussed with all patients. Most people are reluctant to consider long-term medication after a single episode, for several reasons - see consumer resistance in the paragraphs below. Considerations regarding prophylactic therapy include the severity of the initial episode, and the social and financial implications of a recurrence at a particular time if treatment is withdrawn Two or more attacks should strongly support a case for long-term treatment. There is some evidence that prophylactic antidepressant therapy reduces the risk of the illness worsening progressively in the long-term.

Common causes of failure to treat the disease effectively include:

1. The most alarming failure in management is to miss the diagnosis altogether. Because many of the symptoms are somatic (physical symptoms), the underlying mood disorder is commonly missed. For example, studies suggest that 30% of patients develop overt depression after a heart attack, yet only a minority are diagnosed and even fewer, appropriately treated. Is this relevant? Of course! Depression following coronary thrombosis, apart from causing intense psychic suffering, increases the risk of further attacks and shortens life expectancy.

2. The second failure is to treat the illness appropriately. Even if the diagnosis is made and the illness treated with medication, doses are commonly inadequate and given for too short a period to have much impact on the illness.

3. Consumer resistance. The illness has a stigma. Unfortunately, the name suggests a simple episode of misery or sadness. It sounds trivial and is understood as such by the public. The illness affects body and mind, and is associated with demonstrable abnormalities in brain function, but try explaining that to your spouse, your boss or your mother-in-law when you have been too exhausted and

depressed to get out of bed for the last three weeks. The tragedy of this perception is that it leads to prolonged and unnecessary suffering and can, of course, be fatal. Drug therapy is essential for severe depression (melancholia) and should be strongly considered in mild to moderate depression. It is the most effective form of treatment in serious illness (apart from electro-convulsive therapy in a small drug-resistant subgroup), and at least equally effective to therapy by a psychologist in mild to moderate illness.

4.   Drug therapy has had its fair share of bad press. Modern therapy is of considerable help to most sufferers but we still have a way to go in developing better drugs with fewer side-effects. A range of different agents is currently available. The two most commonly used groups are the original antidepressants, the tricyclics, and the newer specific serotonin re-uptake inhibitors (SSRIs). Tricyclics in common usage include amitriptyline, imipramine, nortriptyline and desipramine. Commonly used SSRIs include fluoxetine (Prozac), paroxetine, sertraline, citalopram and fluvoxamine. There are other drug classes, such as the older monoamine uptake inhibitors, and newer agents are becoming available with increasing frequency. Newer drugs include the SNRI (serotonin noradrenaline reuptake inhibitor) venlafaxine, reversible monoamine inhibitors such as moclobemide, and drugs that fall into less well-defined groups such as nefazodone and mirtazapine.

Consumer resistance to drug therapy is reduced if the following facts are clearly explained:

♦   Antidepressant drugs are not addictive. They are not like barbiturates, benzodiazepines or other tranquillisers. People don't break into drugstores to steal the Prozac.

♦   They don't work immediately. They take up to six weeks in adequate dosage to be effective.

♦   An individual drug may have unacceptable side-effects and/or be ineffective in up to 30% of patients. Such patients frequently respond to a drug from another class with a different side-effect profile.

♦ Tolerance to minor side-effects commonly diminishes with time.

♦ The drugs must be prescribed for a minimum of six months. A shorter duration of therapy is almost always followed by relapse.

Doctors commonly fail to prescribe prophylactic antidepressant therapy to patients at high risk for recurrence. Prophylactic therapy should clearly be considered in groups at high risk for relapse, and those to whom a relapse at a particular time would have serious consequences. Long-term maintenance therapy is increasingly recognised as the most important way to control recurrent depressive illness.

Some (notice I said some) forms of psychological therapy are probably as effective as antidepressant therapy for mild to moderate depression, and may have an additive effect when combined with antidepressants. The therapies that come to mind include Cognitive Behaviour Therapy (CBT) and Interpersonal Psychotherapy (IPT). Both forms of therapy should be used for a finite period of time (a month or so). IPT teaches practical problem-solving techniques (a bit like a chat and sympathy with a good friend). CBT identifies individual thinking habits that are dysfunctional. An example is dichotomous thinking - real black and white thinking with no shades of grey. If something is not perfect, it must be absolutely terrible. An idea is either great or appalling. Another example is catastrophising. Your absent-minded boss (thinking of her nubile young personal assistant) forgets to acknowledge you in the hallway so you immediately assume that she hates you and that you are going to be fired in the near future.

The interesting thing about us humans is that we are not remotely like machines. Moods influence thoughts and thoughts influence moods. Depressed mood causes negativistic thinking patterns and vice versa. A vicious cycle ensues and the consequence is an emotional and cognitive downward spiral into a black hole. It is apparent that interruption of the cycle by changing thinking patterns or normalising mood by means of antidepressant drug therapy are both likely to be of value in breaking the depressive cycle. Emotional reasoning is a common form of dysfunctional thinking that can be helped by CBT. The basis of this type of flawed thinking is that if you feel an emotion, then you automatically assume that the underlying premise must be true.

Interestingly, there is also some evidence (class II) that exercise is helpful as adjunctive therapy in relieving mild to moderate depressive symptoms, and may play a role in preventing recurrence. I strongly endorse this.

Folks if you get the illness, remember it is common, it is not a personal failing, and it responds to therapy. I personally would take the soft option, namely the medication, because I am not into therapy. I emphasise again that any form of psychotherapy should be short-term, although the lessons learned should be practised for a lifetime. The Freudian concept of weekly exploration of the subconscious for three decades is certainly financially rewarding to the therapist, but lacks the support of well designed scientific research and is based purely on increasingly outdated theory. It has not been shown to be consistently efficacious in controlled studies.

The ancient Greeks had a most appropriate term for severe depression. They called it melancholia. The direct English translation is "black bile". They believed an accumulation of bile poisoned the body to produce the illness. They were way ahead of us in recognising that depression is a medical illness. Black bile is perhaps the most appropriate name for this horrifying and bewildering affliction, but of course, doesn't do medical jargon justice. Moodstorm or "implosion of the soul" are similarly evocative terms that have been used in an attempt to convey the unbelievable emotional anguish of the condition.

Don't forget all those unnecessary lost QALYs for patients not treated. Depression appears to be more common in women. Have a high level of personal awareness of the symptoms of the condition, ladies, as one in five of you will experience this illness during your lifetime, and the suffering engendered should be largely unnecessary with effective treatment. I'll end this chapter with a poem, which perhaps enhances the understanding of this illness.

Melancholic meltdown

Depression is an endless succession
Of black dawns,
Vacant smiles,
Faded sunsets,
And silent screams
Reverberating
Through long funereal nights
Of inexplicable anguish.

- Depression is one of the major threats to long-term quality existence in the new millennium.
- It is frequently under-diagnosed.
- Unfortunately, the illness still carries a stigma.
- Appropriate therapy is available and usually very effective.
- The disease tends to recur and maintenance therapy should be considered.

* Acknowledgement

The DSM 4 criteria have been reprinted with permission from the *Diagnostic and Statistical Manual of Mental Disorders*, Fourth Edition, Text Revision. © 2000 American Psychiatric Association.

References

1. TYLEE A, WALTERS P. The burden of depression. *Hospital Medicine* 2002; 10: 580-581.
2. American Psychiatric Association. *Diagnostic and Statistical Manual of Mental Disorders*, Fourth Edition, Text Revision. American Psychiatric Association, Washington, DC, 2000.

Chapter 14

Alzheimer's and other brain robbers

The diagnosis of Alzheimer's disease or any other form of dementia is a nightmare which scares most people more than the diagnosis of cancer. No-one wants to lose their marbles. Dementia steals brains and minds. Your mind is the essence of your being. It is you - who you are and how you perceive and interact with the outside world on an intellectual, emotional and spiritual level. It is your most precious asset and the repository of your soul. Cherish, nurture and protect it.

Thanks wiseguy. Enough of the fancy prose and poetry already. I would protect my mind if I could. No-one volunteers for Alzheimer's dementia, you know. You told us that the population was aging. Well, we all know that the incidence of Alzheimer's disease increases with age. You also mentioned that about 45% of people over the age of 80 have dementia of varying degrees of severity. As far as I know, it is not possible to prevent or cure the disease. So what am I supposed to do? Die earlier?

So what causes Alzheimer's and what are the diagnostic criteria? We don't know the cause unfortunately. Brain tissue studies show extracellular neuritic plaques containing amyloid deposits, and neurofibrillary tangles. I agree that this information is hardly helpful to the layman. There is usually no strong hereditary basis for most sufferers from the illness, which is reassuring. Age is a risk factor. Lying about your age doesn't seem to prevent the disease unfortunately. Neither does Botox nor the conventional facelift.

How are we sure that dementia is related to Alzheimer's disease? During life we are not sure. The diagnosis is made after death by post-mortem examination. This is not much help to the patient. In adult patients of advanced age, multiple illnesses can contribute to any dementing disease process. Some of these are treatable. There is a range of diseases similar to Alzheimer's disease that may cause dementia, and which also involve abnormal accumulation of protein in brain tissue. These include Frontotemporoparietal dementia, Multisystem Atrophy, Progressive Supranuclear Palsy (poor old Dudley Moore died from PSP) and advanced Parkinson's disease. Vascular dementia due to multiple strokes (either minor, and individually unnoticed, or major) plays a grossly under-rated role in contributing to dementia in many patients with other clinical diagnoses.

OK, OK, OK. Let's start by defining the clinical signs of dementia. Dementia is a condition in which there is progressive deterioration in memory, speech, reading, writing, intellectual functioning, orientation, problem-solving and insight. Gee, that's one long-winded definition. Let's simplify by describing the individual symptoms.

The slow development of forgetfulness is the first obvious symptom. Day-to-day happenings are not remembered. Items get lost. Appointments are forgotten. Names and seldom-used words go west. Insight into the memory loss is minimal. The patient may have some vague idea that something is wrong but cannot define it. This differs from the memory loss that occurs to all of us as we get older. We recognise this. We are concerned about it and compensate by using reminders like diaries and nagging spouses.

As the illness progresses other defects become more obvious. Speech becomes halting and words or names often cannot be found. Comprehension gradually deteriorates. Writing worsens similarly and reading is abandoned. Arithmetic calculation becomes impaired. Insight deteriorates progressively. Carrying out tasks (like getting dressed, personal hygiene etc.) becomes a problem. As the disease advances, speech can practically disappear and recognition (even of spouse and children) may be lost, which is obviously very distressing for family. Social functioning and behaviour in public becomes a real problem. Loss of visuospatial orientation means that the patient gets lost easily. Loss of diurnal variation occurs. This is often called sundowning. When the sun goes down, the patient gets up to play. Chaos invariably ensues.

In the advanced stages of the illness, the patient may be totally speechless, recognise no-one, be unable to carry out the simplest tasks, and be totally dependent for all activities of daily living.

A case scenario might help clarify the picture more effectively. The family notice that granny is becoming a trifle forgetful at times. She forgets to meet you for tea that has been a routine every Thursday morning for the last 15 years. She appears vague at times. Previously houseproud, she now neglects housework. Forgetfulness increases. Her personal attire and hygiene become erratic. She can't remember the names of recent acquaintances. She doesn't recognise or remember cousins who she hasn't seen for years. Abstemious in the past, she now has a drink or two and gets drunk on small amounts of alcohol. She still drives a car but can't find her way home one afternoon and is taken to the local police station. You are called. At the police station she looks bewildered and is not sure why she is there. A policeman asks her age. She can't remember. You are shocked. She remembers her date of birth and you feel relieved. Phew! She can't be that bad. Then she is asked today's date. She says she isn't sure, but, when pressed, speculates that it is about the tenth of March 1997. Given the fact that it is Christmas Eve, 2002, you realise just how bad things have become. Granny has dementia. She is clearly unemployable now, except maybe as a politician. Furthermore, her intellectual capacity seems pretty borderline for driving a car. Her freedom and mobility are threatened. She is assessed by a physician and admitted to hospital for tests. The scans and psychometric testing confirm moderate dementia. The scan shows some brain shrinkage and "white matter" ischaemic changes. The diagnosis of moderate dementia is made. Granny will not be able to cope at home. She is adamant she does not want to leave her home. This is understandable even in the context of limited insight. In 20 years of medical practice I have yet to be thanked by any patient whom I have committed to rest home care. What is the family to do? A compromise is made. Aunt Ethel, the archetypal family spinster, will move in and care for gran. Aunt Ethel moves in. After a month, gran's condition is unchanged and she seems happy enough, living permanently in March 1997. Aunt Ethel, on the other hand, looks totally wrecked. There is no other word for it. She has been a 24-hr carer seven days a week. Her nights are punctuated by gran bathing and cooking at two in the morning, dressing at 4a.m., and attempting to go walk-about. She is intermittently incontinent. She can be combative and is twice the size of aunt Ethel. Two months later, aunt Ethel's emotional and physical health has deteriorated to such a degree that she is hospitalised for a week. This is a common consequence for long-term carers of Alzheimer's patients. Studies have confirmed that their physical and emotional health is often neglected due to the stress of their other obligations. Social isolation can occur. Few relatives regularly visit because of gran's dementia. She can't be taken to the cinema, the concert, or the debutantes' ball. Gran is institutionalised. She dies eight years later, after ongoing mental and subsequent physical disintegration.

OK, so you thought there was no way to prevent or cure Alzheimer's dementia. Over the last few years we have recognised that making a single diagnosis as to the cause of a dementia is simplistic. Dementia occurs largely in the elderly. As we age, multiple disease processes develop and often act collaboratively in causing disease. For example, we now know that longstanding untreated hypertension doubles the risk of dementia. We also know that small strokes are often clinically unapparent (i.e. cause no symptoms whatsoever) but can insidiously steal your brain, starting with the very expensive piano lessons. This is why control of hypertension is so important. I personally believe that high normal blood pressure (i.e. blood pressure close to the upper end of the normal range), should also be considered an indication for active therapy if there are other risk factors for stroke. We do know from a recent study (the PROGRESS study) that treating patients with a past history of stroke and with no evidence of hypertension reduces the risk of recurrent stroke and improves life expectancy. Treatment of high cholesterol and the use of low-dose aspirin should be considered in patients with any risk of atherosclerosis for the same reasons. A range of diseases work together to bump us off as we get older, and treatment of readily treatable conditions becomes critical in this situation.

And the Alzheimer's? How can we otherwise minimise our risk? The saying "Use it or lose it" is never more relevant than at advanced age. It is critically important to keep using the old brain. Reading, bridge, university courses, work, socialising and living as full a life as possible, are important in maintaining verbal, arithmetic and social skills. Older individuals living in isolation are at increased risk for dementia, and it is thought that the lack of mental and social stimulation accelerates loss of brain function. So use it or lose it folks! Keep active, and mentally and physically fit, even if the physical part does involve popping a few pills. Recent research confirms that the adult human brain contains stem cells that can evolve into new nerve cells. Brain activity stimulates this process. Previous concepts that refused to acknowledge the fact that even old brains can regenerate and produce new brain cells have been largely discredited.

Drug therapy for Alzheimer's disease is, unfortunately, not terribly effective. A group of drugs called anticholinesterases prevent the breakdown of a brain chemical called acetylcholine that is necessary for thinking. Increasing the concentration of acetylcholine can produce mild, short-lived improvement in early Alzheimer's disease. This isn't exactly a cure. It is, I suppose, a start. High doses of vitamin E are perhaps worth trying in early disease but only because we have so little else to offer medicinally. A host of other therapies have been tried without success, including non-steroidal anti-inflammatory drugs and alternative substances such as the well-known ginkgo biloba.

To sum up, multiple conditions probably contribute to the dementia of the elderly. It is important to aggressively treat the things we can. Prophylaxis also involves exercising the mind, as discussed above. Treatment of established dementia is in its infancy, but may be worth trying in patients with early dementia. Current therapy only stabilises the condition in early dementia and for a finite period of time, unfortunately. The trick therefore, is to minimise your risk by exercising your mind. This involves active mind exercise. Watching 10,000 sitcoms a year is not mind exercise. Interact socially. Read. Buy books. Experiment with new ideas and keep learning.

It is important to be aware that reversible causes of dementia do occur and that full medical assesment is mandatory before making the diagnosis. Examples of these reversible causes include hypothyroidism (an underfunctioning thyroid gland) and vitamin B12 deficiency (usually secondary to pernicious anaemia). It goes without saying that a brain scan is necessary as part of the assesment. Brain scans alone cannot make the diagnosis usually, as there is an overlap between the appearance of the normal aging brain and early dementia.

Interestingly, recent evidence strongly implicates cannabis use with the subsequent development of schizophrenia. Up to now the accepted dogma is that cannabis triggers the onset or relapse of schizophrenia in predisposed individuals. These new studies, published in the *BMJ*, indicate that cannabis use is associated with much later development of schizophrenia. So maybe illicit drug use can predispose to permanent brain damage in the long-term. We know that some licit drug use, eg. four pints of Scotch daily for 30 years, certainly increases dementia risk. So all of us who floated through the '70s on a cloud (if you will pardon the expression) and think we are Napoleon, are probably not.

Depression can mimic dementia and is also important to exclude before attaching labels to patients.

- Dementia must be investigated to exclude treatable causes.
- Mental fitness must be maintained to reduce dementia risk.
- Treatment of hypertension and other risk factors for stroke reduce dementia risk.
- Drug therapy for Alzheimer's disease has mild benefit early in the illness.

References

1. RITCHIE K, LOVESTONE S. The dementias. *The Lancet* 2002; 360: 1759-66.
2. REY JM. Cannabis and mental health. *BMJ* 2002; 325: 1183-1184.
3. VALLES FERNANDEZ MN *et al.* Health and social problems of caregivers of patients with dementia. *Aten Primaria* 1998; 22(8): 481-5.
4. DONALDSON C, TARRIER N, BURNS A. Determinants of carer stress in Alzheimer's disease. *Int J Geriatr Psychiatry* 1998; 13(4): 248-56.
5. SHUMACHER SA *et al.* Estrogen plus progestin and the incidence of dementia and mild cognitive impairment in post-menopausal women. *JAMA* 2003; 289 No. 20.
6. SANO M *et al.* A controlled trial of Selegiline, Alpha-Tocopherol, or both as treatment of Alzheimer's disease. *NEJM* 1997; 1336: 1216-22.

Chapter 15

The dreadful truth about statistics

In the last chapter I emphasised brain stimulation. Well, this is the chapter where it happens. So put down that gin and tonic immediately and concentrate. Until the mid 20th century, medical journal articles were largely biased, subjective guesstimates based on anecdotes (quaint medical stories based on survival, or otherwise, of individual patients). Attempts to validate studies in a measurable scientific way were introduced at that time. Many subsequent studies still had major methodological problems. This means they weren't really valid when subjected to rigorous statistical scrutiny. Furthermore, researchers often had serious conflicts of interest. Drug companies, who clearly had a vested interest in the outcomes, commonly sponsored studies. Study results that never supported the use of the particular company's trial drug were commonly disregarded. Fly me around the world first class and treat me like a king, and I suspect I might be susceptible to bias. What can I say? I am only human. Conflicts of interest were not declared. Negative studies were seldom published. Which drug company wants to advertise to the world that its new wonder product is no better than noodle soup? From the point of view of medical journals trying to survive in a competitive market, this is understandable. Imagine newspaper headlines declaring that absolutely nothing of note has happened in the last 24 hours. The paper emphasising a general lack of excitement and no new happenings would struggle to survive. No-one wants to publish an article declaring an absence of any relationship between migraine and anal warts. Similarly, an article emphasising that Prince Whoever has spent a quiet weekend without making sexual overtures to the children's nanny does not attract attention. This is called publication bias. Excitement is the name of the game for editors. Positive results that challenge current dogma or claim important medical breakthroughs sell journals. The obvious consequence is a serious publication bias in favour of studies that show benefits. Situational bias is also common. Preselect your study group and the outcome can be virtually guaranteed.

Yip. Even now we are struggling to address these issues. Researchers are now expected to declare any conflict of interest. If researcher A finds product A is wonderful, it is helpful to know if researcher A has received any gifts or shares from Company A. Retrospective analysis of many medical studies in the '60s, '70s and '80s, confirm that conflicts of interest were a serious problem. So-called scientific publications were biased. The medication often didn't work. At least we are now attempting to address the issue robustly, but concern over publication bias, in particular, remains. Negative results are unexciting. The fire brigade was quiet today. No fires have been reported and no cats were stuck up trees. There were no sex scandals. No politician seduced his secretary or accepted bribes. No choirboys were molested. You get my drift. Boring, boring, boring. The same situation exists in the scientific world. Sorry guys but there were no dramatic medical breakthroughs today.

Statistics can be even more misleading. Imagine two patients, Mr. A and Mr. B, both suffering from identical cancers of the widget. Both patients will die in nine years. There is no effective treatment for cancer of the widget. Neither patient is aware that they are suffering from cancer of the widget because the disease is in an early asymptomatic phase. The cancer of the widget will only cause symptoms in eight years time. A year after the onset of symptoms, both patients will die irrespective of any treatment. Both patients are middle-aged men who won the lotto two years ago. They are now very wealthy and suffering from a mid-life crisis. The obvious consequence is a new 22 year old blond wife for each of these men. They feel well. Actually, to be honest, as a result of the introduction of Viagra, they are both having the time of their lives. Until now, there has been no screening test for early asymptomatic cancer of the widget.

Company X develops a screening test to identify early cancer of the widget. Mr. A goes for screening and to his horror discovers he has cancer. Several treatments are available. No treatment has been scientifically proven to cure the cancer or prolong life. One form of treatment involves chopping off the widget. The second form of therapy involves frying the widget with radiotherapy. Mr A elects to undergo removal of his widget. This has an 80% risk of permanent impotence. Bit of a tragedy really, as the new wife's attributes are largely physical. Anyway, he has the surgery, loses the new wife and most of the lotto money, and dies nine years later. Mr. B does not undergo screening for cancer of the widget. His disease presents eight years later and he dies a year after onset of the symptoms. Man, did he have fun in the interim. So what conclusion do the researchers come to? The researchers say that early diagnosis of cancer of the widget with appropriate treatment prolongs life by eight years. Remember Mr. A lived nine years after detection of his illness by screening. Admittedly the treatment was mutilating. Mr. B only lived one year after diagnosis of his cancer. You and I know that Mr. A and Mr. B both had identical life expectancies. The screening program however, suggests improved life expectancy with early diagnosis by screening. It is obvious this is pure drivel. This type of bias is called lead-time bias. In the above example, early diagnosis appeared to improve life expectancy when in this situation it obviously had no benefit, and, in fact, had serious disadvantages.

Next we come to length-time bias. Mr. C And Mr. D both undergo an annual screening test to detect early asymptomatic cancer of the widget. Not all cancers of the widget are the same. Mr. C is lucky enough to have a very slow-growing cancer of the widget that will take 25 years to become symptomatic and 30 years to kill him. In fact, his cancer is growing so slowly that he is far more likely to die from other disease rather than the cancer. Mr. D has a very aggressive cancer that develops over one week and kills the patient three days later. Annual screening is thus far more likely to detect the slow-growing cancer of Mr. C than the rapidly growing cancer of Mr. D. In other words, screening is more likely to detect slow-growing, less severe forms of cancer than rapidly growing cancers which produce symptoms early. This can overestimate the value of screening. In this situation, screening for cancer appears to improve life expectancy because of length-time bias. Garbage in; garbage out.

There are a large number of ways in which studies can be flawed. Flaws are not always easy to identify, even for researchers. It is critical that expert statisticians are involved in the formulation of any study to minimise the potential for bias. A well-known study on human sexuality was widely accepted as gospel (if you will pardon the expression) for decades, in spite of major limitations in the design process. A simple analogy may be helpful in demonstrating defects in apparently basic aspects of study design, such as questionnaire development. Suppose there was a question on bestiality. Proponents of the practice are hardly likely to answer honestly. And a question on impotence? By a sexy young female researcher? Denial will almost certainly distort the responses. Homosexuality? This is part of the normal range of human sexuality but is still emotionally charged. If questions are deemed extreme or inappropriate by much of a society, then most of the study sample tends to ignore the study. Response rates tend to be low. Only extremists who feel particularly strongly about a particular proposition respond, producing nonsense results where only the extremist viewpoints are reflected. If these are then assumed to reflect the normal pattern of behaviour in society, we end up with ridiculous data. Garbage in; garbage out. When highly emotive issues such as human sexuality are involved, the results become patently absurd.

Studies measure probability. The basic approach is to estimate the likelihood that a particular outcome could have happened purely due to chance. The probability value (p value) cut off is usually 0.05 or less. A value of 0.05 means that the probability that the results could be due to chance is 5% or less. Obviously sample sizes, study design, exclusion criteria and a load of other stuff so beloved by nerds (sorry biostaticians), are crucial to meaningful study design.

Confounding bias is a common problem. Until recently we thought hormone replacement therapy reduced the risk of heart attack and stroke. "Healthy user" and "compliance" biases were subsequently recognised as causing significant bias. The basic problem was that women on HRT were more likely to be middle class, to see their doctor regularly, and to have other medical conditions recognised and appropriately treated. Comparing these patients to people not using such therapy was invalid because the patient populations were totally dissimilar.

As mentioned in the Introduction, we place great importance on classes or grades of evidence. These are graded according to the quality of study design, the number of studies of similar quality producing the same outcome etc. Class I evidence strongly supports a particular course of action; class II evidence is less rigorous and so on. A particular expert's opinion, unsupported by scientific research, is class IV at best. Thus when an 88 year old retired doctor makes outrageous claims regarding his baldness/impotence/haemorrhoid cure, caution is required. The evidence is suspect.

Other terms can be exploited to make a product sound far more effective (or hazardous) than it really is. Consider products A and B. Product A is ten times more effective than product B in treating cancer of the widget. However, product A doubles your risk for a fatal heart attack when compared to product B. In other words product B carries 50% of the risk of heart attack when compared to product A. In statistical terms, the relative risk reduction for fatal heart attack when using product B is 50%. The risk is halved. Sounds worrying, doesn't it? Which product will you use? You need information that is often not supplied, either in order to sensationalise the issue, or to promote product B. The information required is the absolute risk reduction in fatal heart attack when using product B. If the risk of having a fatal heart attack when using product A is 1 in 10 million, the risk using product B, is 50% of that, which is 1 in 20 million. Thus the absolute increase in risk of a fatal heart attack when using product A is minute. So even though your chances of fatal heart attack are doubled, your real risk remains negligible when using product A. If product A is a life-saving drug, the failure to use it because of deliberately misleading statistics is criminal. Not only the public and the lay media, but also the medical media and profession can be misled if statistical issues are not scrupulously assessed. This will remain a common problem as drug advertising to the lay public becomes more prevalent.

Much of what I have described above, might sound a bit like gobbledegook. I have included it in the book to emphasise the complexity of statistical design necessary to produce sound scientific research. What I am trying to say is that there is enormous scope for nonsense research out there; the pressures to publish are enormous, there are commonly major vested interests involved, and that if you search for long enough you will find something to support practically any point of view. In my view, Class I evidence (unequivocally proven) is the ideal class required if a doctor expects an asymptomatic patient to swallow a pill for the next 30 years.

Many books aimed at the lay market quote large numbers of studies in their reference section. It is impossible for a layperson to be able to evaluate the validity of these. It is common in this type of literature for poor studies to be quoted to support and promote a particular viewpoint, even when the best medical evidence suggests otherwise. Conspiracy theories about orchestrated movements of conventional medicine to destroy the credibility of a particular practitioner who has discovered the one true diet, impotency medication, or food supplement that flies in the face of current dogma, are not uncommonly used by non-mainstream practitioners. Valid complaints in this situation are very rare. Sorry folks, I know that is disappointing to some people. But it is true.

Alternative medicine has not fully embraced the concept of scientific proof, so to be honest, there is little out there to reassure patients regarding safety or efficacy. Fortunately, most users of alternative medicines or supplements tend to be healthy, so lack of true efficacy is not such a big deal, particularly if there is a strong placebo effect (placebo - as mentioned before, if you believe it is good for you, then it is good for you i.e. confers some benefit). As mentioned earlier in the book, I am not knocking alternative medicine overall.

Searching the Internet for information about medical topics has major limitations, unless the quality of the information can be verified as high. There are a large number of sites available to the profession. Reading about a disease can be counter-productive if the information contained is controversial or not relevant to a particular clinical context. Nevertheless, the days of medical arrogance are over.

Two useful sites are the Cochrane collaboration website and the National Library of Medicine site.

Cochrane collaboration website URL:
http://www.cochrane.org/

NLM website URL:
http://www.ncbi.nlm.nih.gov/PubMed/

Go on. Get in there and have some fun. Then torment your doctor with your extensive medical knowledge. And by the way, you are the most important final arbiter of any decisions pertaining to any medical treatment you may require. So learn about your illness if it is likely to be a chronic problem. And take what material you have found to your consultation, if you have relevant concerns. It will keep the doctor on her toes.

● Statistical research can produce false outcomes if poorly structured.

● Good measurable research remains the only way to move forward in evaluating the benefits or otherwise, of various treatments.

● Care should be based on the best available evidence.

References

1.   COCHRANE COLLABORATION http://www.cochrane.org/.

2.   LEXCHIN J *et al.* Pharmaceutical industry sponsorship and research outcome and quality: systemic review. *BMJ* 2003; 326: 1167-70.

Chapter 16

Hormone replacement therapy or not?

Hormone Replacement Therapy (HRT) has had a tough time of late. Women live about eight years longer than men on average. Ischaemic heart disease, the biggest killer, is just as common in post-menopausal women as in men, but is rare before menopause. There are theoretical reasons why female hormones (oestrogen and progestin) might reduce the risk for ischaemic heart disease and stroke, principally by exerting a favourable effect on blood HDL cholesterol (the good guy). HRT also increases bone density, thereby reducing the risk of osteoporosis. Osteoporosis dramatically increases the risk for fracture and HRT has been prescribed to maintain bone mineral density in post-menopausal women, until recently. There is fair evidence that use of HRT does reduce fracture rates in older women. There is some evidence to suggest that HRT also reduces colorectal cancer risk.

Of more immediate importance to most women who use this therapy is the prevention of the distressing symptoms of menopause. These include hot flushes, vaginal dryness and discomfort during intercourse, stress incontinence, and perhaps low grade depressive symptoms.

Now as it turns out, HRT appears not to be as safe as we thought it was. HRT does not reduce the risk of heart attack and stroke. In fact, there is fair to good evidence that HRT can increase heart attack and stroke risk. It certainly increases the risk for a second event in heart attack survivors. It definitely increases the risk of breast cancer and venous thromboembolism (blood clots in the legs, as in the recently named economy class syndrome). A recent study revealed that HRT probably slightly increases dementia risk in older women, presumably by increasing the risk of stroke. The individual risk is small and was probably overlooked in the past because of the "healthy user" bias. There is insufficient scientific evidence at present to recommend for or against HRT to prevent ovarian cancer. The impact on mortality from breast cancer or cardiovascular causes is currently unclear. What about those women who have had a hysterectomy and are thus able to use oestrogen without progestin because of the absence of problems pertaining to vaginal bleeding? (Oestrogen and progestin are usually combined and taken continuously to reduce problems of vaginal bleeding). There is no clear evidence one way or another, regarding the routine use of oestrogen for disease prevention in this group.

OK then, I hear you ask, "Why do women live longer than men?" I would have thought the answer is obvious. God is a woman. But I digress. The real issue is how individual women make decisions regarding personal use of HRT. The US Preventive Services Task Force conclude that the harmful effects of oestrogen and progestin are likely to exceed the chronic disease prevention benefits in most women. This simply means that HRT should not be used as standard long-term therapy in all post-menopausal women for the prevention of disease, as the risks are likely to outweigh the benefits for most. Does this mean it should never be used? If it is used, is there a safe duration of use? Or will bearded women with vaginal dryness become the post-menopausal norm in the 21st century?

Let's look at the problem from a more realistic perspective. The absolute increase in risk of HRT to any one individual is small. Furthermore, not all women are at equal risk for the various conditions ascribed to HRT. There may in fact, be subgroups who might benefit from HRT. An example would be a woman at major risk of osteoporosis and colorectal cancer and at very low personal risk of breast cancer or cardiovascular disease. Multiple studies have been undertaken to evaluate HRT. Apart from two quality studies using daily conjugated oestrogen and progestin, the design and formulation of the studies has been of variable quality. In different studies, HRT was administered in different dosages and formulations. Even conjugated equine oestrogen has different uptake rates in different individuals, depending on how the liver handles the drug. It may be that there are formulations that are effective and more research needs to be done. So what is the average absolute increase in risk for a lady in the first throes of menopause? The Women's Health Initiative study suggests that for women aged between 50 and 79, for every 10,000 women taking combined oestrogen and progestin therapy for one year, we might expect seven additional heart attacks, eight more strokes, eight more pulmonary emboli and eight more invasive breast cancers. On the upside there would be five fewer hip fractures and six less cancers of the bowel. If you work out the numbers it is obvious that individual risk of a serious adverse event is low, but not non-existent. What is a girl to do? Choices need to be individualised. HRT should not be prescribed for disease prevention. The increased risk of breast cancer does not seem to be a major issue for the first few years of HRT. Current cautious recommendations are that HRT may be used for treatment of menopausal symptoms for a finite period (1-2 years) and in as low a dose as possible, provided there are no personal contra-indications to such treatment. But watch this space ladies, as the last word on HRT has yet to be written. And avoid facial hair - it detracts from your personality.

- HRT is not the universal panacea for a longer healthier life after menopause.
- There is a small but definite increase in risk of several diseases with HRT therapy.
- The current conservative approach would be to recommend HRT for control of menopausal symptoms for a restricted period of time.

References

1. U.S. Preventive Services Task Force. Postmenopausal Hormone Replacement Therapy for Primary Prevention of Chronic Conditions: Recommendations and Rationale. *Annals of Internal Medicine* 2002; 137 (No 10): 834-839.
2. JOSEFSON D. Latest HRT trial results show risk of dementia. *BMJ* 2003; 326(7401): 1232.

Chapter 17

Screening for cancer of the breast

I am starting this chapter with the definition of cure for any illness. A cure may be defined not only as the eradication of a disease process, but also as the complete restoration of health, including the physical, emotional, spiritual, intellectual and sexual aspects. For too long the narrow definition of cure implied eradication of a disease process only. The devastating side-effects of such "cures" were often appalling. Eradication of a disease process alone is hardly a cure in a truly holistic sense. If doctors understood this more clearly, the approach to disease eradication may have been less barbarous than it sometimes has been in the past. Past management of breast disease is an excellent example of the limitations inherent in regarding cure as disease eradication only.

Cancer of the breast is the commonest cause of cancer in women (excluding skin cancers). In the year 2000, about 185,000 cases of invasive breast cancer and 42,000 breast cancer-related deaths occurred in the USA. Breast cancer mortality is decreasing in women and it is not the commonest cause of cancer-related death in females. That dubious honour goes to lung cancer, largely because lung cancer has such a high case fatality rate. Eighty-six percent of patients who present with lung cancer are dead within five years. Breast cancer, of course, has a whole range of emotional implications poorly understood by the male of the species. Original therapies involved radical and mutilating surgery, which was thought necessary to eradicate the cancer. The so-called cured were commonly emotionally devastated in terms of their perception of their sexuality, their completeness as women, and the consequences to personal sexual relationships. These issues still exist, but encouraging developments in terms of screening have had a significant impact in terms of early detection of disease. Furthermore, there is now good evidence that removal of the tumour instead of the entire breast does not increase the risk of recurrence. The need for surgical treatment or radiotherapy to axillary lymph nodes (the glands in the armpit) has been more clearly defined and is limited to a smaller subgroup now. Long-term consequences of this procedure (in particular, a persistently swollen arm due to lymphoedema i.e. tissue fluid accumulation), are thus now relatively infrequent.

What is your individual risk? Approximately 10% of human breast cancers have a familial (hereditary) basis. A number of genes have been implicated in these hereditary cases. In normal circumstances, these genes control cell growth and repair damage to genetic material. Do you as an individual need to have some sort of genetic screening for these? Yes, if there is a strong family history of the disease. The genes involved in different mutations include the p53 tumour suppressor gene, and the BRCA-1 and BRCA-2 genes. Genetic testing is readily available and enables early decisions to be made about long-term strategies for disease prevention. The BRCA-1 gene mutation, for example, is associated with a 60-80% lifetime risk for breast cancer and a 33% risk of ovarian cancer. The BRCA-2 gene appears to be associated with an increased risk of breast cancer in men and women. So the message here is to ensure that you have access to genetic screening if you have a strong family history of breast cancer.

OK, so 10% of breast cancers are inherited. The remaining 90% occur sporadically i.e. out of the blue. Breast cancer is a hormone dependant disease. If you've never had ovaries and never received oestrogen replacement therapy, your chances of acquiring the disease are very low. This applies essentially to all men (excluding the occasional transvestite).

Big help for most women. Also the longer the duration of oestrogen exposure, the higher the risk. Women with early menarche (onset of menstruation) and late menopause are at higher lifetime risk. Not much you can do about that either. Increased body mass seems to be associated with increased risk of breast cancer but the role of specific dietary components is unproven. There is a correlation between alcohol consumption and breast cancer. Moderate alcohol consumption marginally increases absolute risk of breast cancer. Far more women die from heart disease and stroke, where moderate alcohol intake decreases risk, so the net result favours moderate alcohol consumption to prolong life. Thank

God for that. Not bad to have a medication that works, and makes your spouse appear more attractive at the same time, ladies. We know that HRT seems to double the risk for breast cancer as discussed previously.

For women at average risk of breast cancer, there are a number of reasonable recommendations to enable early disease detection. The first is monthly self-examination of the breasts (a reasonably knowledgeable and enthusiastic partner might suffice). It is sensible. Have your physician demonstrate the technique. The potential spin-off is early diagnosis of cancer, which can be reasonably expected to increase the likelihood of cure.

A recent journal article suggested that monthly self-examination of the breasts doesn't improve long-term outcomes, but I wouldn't change my recommendation at this stage. As a compromise, let's insist that your sex partner does the exam. Even without the cancer screening benefit, your love life should get a boost. Furthermore, the smaller any cancer is when detected, the better the chances of limiting surgery to lumpectomy (excising the tumour only) with preservation of the breast.

Physician examination of the breasts is a routine part of every complete physical exam, but is not uncommonly neglected, not because of deliberate negligence but because of the medico-legal risks of breast exam without a chaperone. I would recommend monthly self-examination, annual mammography and annual examination by your physician for all women over the age of 40. There is fair to good evidence that screening mammography can reduce breast cancer deaths by up to 50%. Mammography is by no means a perfect screening tool. It can overlook small cancers and false positive results are not uncommon. Obviously, false positive results (i.e. a mammographic suggestion of cancer in its absence) can be emotionally distressing, but on balance I would still favour screening. A false positive result doesn't mean some misogynist removes the breast. Standard protocols are followed and most patients undergo aspiration biopsy by fine needle rather than chopping out the lump. I won't discuss treatment of breast cancer, or the use of prophylaxis (tamoxifen, raloxifene, aromatase inhibitors or prophylactic mastectomy) in high-risk women, as these complex issues are confined to a small subgroup who clearly need subspecialist input. It is not uncommon for high-risk patients to overestimate their individual risk, and objective decisions about how best to manage patients with a strong hereditary risk for breast cancer remain controversial. Drugs such as tamoxifen and newer agents certainly seem to reduce breast cancer risk in high-risk patients

---

● Breast cancer screening improves early detection rates and outcomes over the age of 40.

References

1. FEIG SA. The current status of screening mammography. *Obstet Gynecol Clin North Am* 2002; 29(1): 123-36.
2. CUZICK J *et al.* Overview of the main outcomes in breast-cancer prevention trials. *The Lancet* 2003; 361: 296-300.

Chapter 18

Women's other bits
Screening for gynaecological malignancies

Let's start with ovarian cancer. This is the leading cause of death from gynaecological cancer in the western world. The disease is less common than breast, lung, and colorectal cancer in women but, unfortunately, tends to be asymptomatic until fairly advanced, so cure is less likely. Early disease is commonly curable by conventional therapy. This is thus a classic cancer presentation where an effective screening test that reliably detects early asymptomatic disease would be extremely valuable. Unfortunately, an accurate, sensitive test that does not produce false positive rates, i.e. a test very specific for ovarian cancer, does not exist. Vaginal examination is a poor screening procedure for early disease. Pelvic ultrasound, using a scanner in contact with the skin of the lower abdomen, is not accurate enough to detect early disease. Transvaginal ultrasound, which is performed by inserting the ultrasound probe into the vagina, picks up early disease more accurately but has a high incidence of false positive results. This is a real problem because further investigation requires laparoscopy or laparotomy. These are substantial and invasive operations with the potential for serious side-effects. Furthermore, they are not cheap. In one study, 67 diagnostic operations were required to diagnose one ovarian cancer. In this situation, the consequences of using a screening program are probably worse than no screening at all. Damn!

What about blood tests? CA-125, a chemical often produced by ovarian cancers, can be measured in the blood and has been tried as a screening tool. Unfortunately, other conditions can elevate CA-125 and the false positive rate in early cancer is too high to make this an effective screening tool. The levels in the blood are often normal in early curable cancer, which means that the test is not sensitive enough to be generally helpful.

Other screening modalities are currently undergoing investigation. Currently, screening is not of proven value among the general population with no known risk factors.

It may be reasonable to screen women with a strong hereditary risk for carcinoma of the ovary. For example, women with the BRCA-1 mutation have a 33% lifetime risk for ovarian cancer. There are a number of other cancer syndromes that are hereditary (see chapter on colorectal cancer) and which may warrant screening for ovarian cancer. Unfortunately, the high false positive rates for screening mean that these patients will also be at risk of unnecessary diagnostic surgery. This is an area that requires complex decision-making, involving both patient and specialist. I would recommend several different opinions before embarking on any course of action.

Next we come to that old nemesis, cancer of the cervix. Rare in nuns, cervical cancer is essentially a long-term consequence of infection with some types of a virus known as Human Papillomavirus. This virus is transmitted sexually. For this reason, risk is increased by the number of lifetime sexual partners. Several subtypes predispose to longstanding infection that can evolve into cancer over a period of years. What is particularly important is that the disease evolves through a premalignant phase during which the patient has no symptoms, but subtle abnormalities develop in the cells of the cervix. The abnormalities are defined as cervical intraepithelial neoplasia (CIN). There are various grades of severity of CIN. A Pap smear can usually detect these cellular abnormalities. Cancer of the cervix used to be the number one fatal malignancy in women, but because of the widespread introduction of screening programs (Yip, using our old friend, the Pap smear), the disease is now largely preventable, or at least curable at an early stage. As a result, it is now way down on the list of malignancies that kill women. See, sometimes us white-coated jerks do make a difference!

Initial screening for this cancer involves the use of the Pap smear, as mentioned above. Recommendations vary but the most prudent approach is perhaps to have yearly smears after the age of 20 or, alternatively, annually after the onset of sexual activity. A single Pap smear can miss cancer. The false negative rate varies. Paradoxically, the smear is most sensitive in the early premalignant phase where a single smear should pick up 90% of cases. Because the disease develops slowly, annual screening remains safe in the investigation of women without abnormal gynaecological symptoms. Serial annual smears dramatically reduce the long-term risk of missing early asymptomatic cancer. As full-blown cancer develops, ulceration, inflammation, and bleeding make the interpretation of the slides more difficult and the false negative rate rises. Thus a Pap smear is not the answer once the patient has symptoms, or if an abnormality of the cervix is obvious by direct colposcopic examination. Colposcopic-directed biopsy is mandatory whenever any abnormality is obvious on the cervix.

OK, what should your expectations be? Use the screening program. Fifty percent of patients with cervical cancer have either never had a Pap smear or not within the last ten years. Patients at the highest risk for cervical cancer are the least likely to be tested regularly. Remember too that doctors sometimes get things wrong (Yip. We never used to know this until the legal profession discharged its moral opportunity to get really rich). Pap smears DO have a false negative rate. Thus they do need to be performed regularly. IF you develop symptoms of abnormal vaginal bleeding, a Pap smear is not adequate as a diagnostic tool. See your gynaecologist for cervical examination. If you are at high risk, i.e. if you had loads of fun during a misspent youth (like me), the importance of screening is crucial. NO-ONE should die from cancer of the cervix now. Vaccines against Human Papillomavirus are currently undergoing trials. If they are effective in preventing infection, cancer of the cervix may become totally preventable by vaccination in the medium-term future.

Cancer of the uterus is the most common gynaecological malignancy. About 36,000 cases of uterine cancer were diagnosed in 1996. About 75% are confined to the body of the uterus so most can be cured. As a result, uterine cancer is only the seventh leading cause of cancer death in females. Ninety percent of cases occur post-menopausally. Most patients present with abnormal symptoms. These include post-menopausal bleeding, and abnormal vaginal discharge. Unfortunately, there are no effective and accurate screening tests. It is thus pretty important to identify if you are at risk, and that you have a high level of awareness about the common presenting symptoms.

Risk factors include:

♦ Obesity - this increases risks 3 to 10 times (Damn! Back to the diet chapter).

♦ Unopposed oestrogen replacement therapy i.e. HRT without progestogen.

♦ Late menopause.

♦ Polycystic ovarian syndrome (PCOS). If you haven't heard of it, you probably haven't got it. PCOS is discussed in more detail in chapter 28.

♦ Irregular, scanty or absent periods.

♦ Tamoxifen - used for treatment (and sometimes for prevention) of breast cancer.

The main symptoms are vaginal bleeding after the menopause and abnormal vaginal discharge. These both need investigation by your gynaecologist. Pap smears are unreliable in diagnosis. Transvaginal ultrasonography also doesn't cut the mustard because of false positive and false negative results. Endometrial biopsy or aspiration are done in the doctor's rooms but are positive in only 80-90% of cases. This means that negative results do not definitively exclude cancer and a formal dilatation and curettage needs to be done under general anaesthetic.

● Screening for cancer of the cervix is mandatory.

● Effective reliable screening tests for ovarian and endometrial cancer do not exist at this stage.

References

1. Screening for cervical cancer: recommendations and rationale. *Am Fam Physician* 2003; 67(8): 1759-66. No authors listed.

2. URBAN N. Specific keynote: ovarian cancer risk assessment and the potential for early detection. *Gynecol Oncol* 2003; 88(1 Pt 2): S75-79.

3. SONODA Y. Optimal therapy and management of endometrial cancer. *Expert Rev Anticancer Ther* 2003; 3(1): 37-47.

Chapter 19

What to do about prostate cancer screening and management

Screening for cancer of the prostate has become a highly controversial issue in the past decade. Prior to this time no sensitive and specific test was available to screen for the problem. Hence the approach to management was at least simplified by the fact that malignancy had usually been diagnosed as a consequence of urinary symptoms. These include urinary infections, difficulty in initiating micturition, poor urinary stream, post-urination dribbling, and the frequent urge to urinate. Of course, these symptoms are usually the presenting symptoms of benign enlargement of the prostate (BPH), which becomes increasingly common as men age. Before you panic I would like to assure you that in most cases, these symptoms are related to BPH and not to prostatic cancer. Delightful, isn't it? Who on earth needs a larger prostate with age? It's not as if we use it as much. Which brings me to my next question - what the hell is the prostate gland, where does it live and what does it do?

The prostate gland is situated in the pelvis just below and adjacent to the bladder, the internal urinary sphincter (this is partly responsible for control of urination), the rectum (your backside), and nerve groupings including those responsible for controlling urination and erections. The normal prostate gland is about the size of a walnut and weighs about 30g. What does it do? It secretes prostatic fluid. The fluid contains constituents that protect and promote the functional properties of the spermatozoa (the sperm cells). It thus plays an essential role in male fertility. Unfortunately, with aging it can become a damned nuisance or worse. The prostate increases in size with age in most men. Certain race groups (such as Caucasians) are more likely to develop benign prostate enlargement (BPH). Male hormone (testosterone - the remarkable chemical that changes that irritating young girl next door into a creature infinitely more interesting during adolescence) plays a role in this enlargement. The prostate gland surrounds the urethra, the pipe connecting the bladder to the outside world. The gland has three zones: a central zone, a transitional zone and a peripheral zone. Because it surrounds the urethra, enlargement can cause obstruction to urinary flow and bingo! All of a sudden you are stuck with the signs described in the first paragraph above. No matter how much you shake and dance, the last drop always falls into your underpants. The longer you live, the more likely you are to experience these symptoms. There are medical and surgical options available for the treatment of BPH. Symptoms do not necessarily worsen over time. The surgical procedure (most commonly a transurethral resection of the prostate) for BPH is far less radical than that for prostatic cancer and serious long-term side-effects are hence far less likely. BPH does not increase the subsequent risk of prostate cancer.

In the last couple of decades or so, Prostate Specific Antigen (PSA) measurement in the blood has become available. This is a reasonably sensitive and specific marker for prostate cancer. Note well that I said reasonably! PSA is a protein normally found in prostatic fluid that helps to maintain the liquid state of the ejaculate. The PSA can be elevated in other conditions such as inflammation of the prostate. A normal PSA does not exclude very early prostate cancer. As mentioned previously, screening should be of value in any cancer that has a long period before symptoms develop, that is curable if detected early (particularly during this presymptomatic period), and which is fatal if diagnosed late. And this is where things start getting complicated.

We need more information about prostate cancer, don't we? Prostate cancer is the commonest cancer in men and the second commonest cause of cancer-related mortality. The commonest cause of cancer-related death in men is lung cancer, because of the high case fatality rate, as mentioned previously.

There seems to be some hereditary contribution, as a significant family history among first-degree relatives doubles the risk. It is commonest in the USA (perhaps due to increased screening) and least common amongst Asian males. Asians who move to the US have their risk increased to the level of other Americans in one generation, so lifestyle factors and diet seem to be important. A high intake of animal fat is suggested statistically as a risk factor. At the end of the day however, there do not seem to be any major preventative factors that can be used to reduce your risk apart from moving to Asia and becoming a vegetarian. Far too radical an option for me.

OK, so far, so good. The vast majority of prostate cancers occur over the age of 50 and routine annual digital rectal examinations (DRE) and PSA measurements have been widely used to detect early cancer. This sounds logical in a hypothetical sense. Surely the earlier a cancer is detected, the greater the possibility of cure.

Unfortunately, it isn't all that simple. Prostate cancer is by nature very variable in its behaviour. Many of the cancers never produce any clinical problems and are found incidentally, either by screening or at post-mortem following death for other reasons. In some patients an aggressive course is followed, whereas, in others, the disease can remain asymptomatic with minimal progression over three or so decades. If 50-year-old men with a 25-year life expectancy are routinely screened, 42% will be found to have microscopic evidence of prostatic cancer; only about 10% will develop symptoms from the cancer during their life; and only 3% will die from it.

Does screening save lives? Well, the jury is still out on that one. Screening has yet to be proven to improve prognosis i.e. life expectancy. A review in the *American Journal of Medicine* in December 2002 expresses strong concerns regarding the widespread use of screening in the absence of meaningful evidence of its value. If a patient is encouraged to undergo screening, an abnormal result almost always creates a situation of positive reinforcement where the patient is grateful for early detection and hence encouraged to undergo treatment. This is a major concern particularly when we examine the nature of prostate cancer and the statistical biases inherent in screening. Remember length-time and lead-time bias. Low-grade tumours that are very slow-growing, and therefore less life-threatening, are far more likely to be picked up by screening. Screening also creates a lead-time bias, where early diagnosis increases length of life (life expectancy) after making the diagnosis, simply because the diagnosis was made early as a result of screening. This falsely suggests that any treatment improves life expectancy, whether this is the case or not. Thus multiple problems exist related to the validity of screening procedures.

Curative therapy (yet to be proven to prolong life expectancy) is offered to men with prostate cancer localised to the gland and with a life expectancy of greater than ten years. It has been suggested (not proven) that these chaps are more likely to die from the cancer than any other cause. The consequences for a substantial number of patients would not be so devastating if the surgery was easy to perform, with minimal risk of death or long-term side-effects. And therein lies a major problem. You will recall that I mentioned that the prostate is very close anatomically to the nerves responsible for promoting erections and preventing urinary incontinence. Radical surgery to the prostate is fraught with risk of damaging these nerves. The downstream consequences (no pun intended) are not funny. No erections without the use of a range of mostly distressing interventions (yes, even if you are a masochist), and permanent incontinence are hardly likely to make you lover of the month. Can we apply percentages to these side-effects? At least 50% (and probably far, far more, if one recognises the biases inherent in such a question) of patients are rendered permanently impotent following curative surgery for cancer of the prostate. Incontinence levels seem to be about 8% or a little less in most series. The mortality with modern surgical techniques is probably less than 1%.

OK then, what about radiotherapy? External beam radiotherapy appears to be as effective as surgery in patients with localised prostate cancer. Another radiotherapy option involves the insertion of radioactive material into the gland itself. This is called brachytherapy. The cancers can be classified according to a variety of systems to identify patients in whom intervention is thought to be of benefit. Disease-free survival for clinically localised prostate cancer after surgery or radiotherapy ranges between 43% and 66%. Radiotherapy causes inflammation of the rectum with bleeding, rectal urgency (got to get to the John real fast or else, with no room for negotiation) and occasionally, rectal incontinence. In general, the incidence of side-effects does appear to be lower and the impotence rate has been reported to be about half that of surgery.

Remember lead- and length-time bias when evaluating results. We don't know whether we should screen, when or whether we should intervene and what to do. Go to a radiotherapist and X-ray therapy is what you are going to get. Go to a surgeon and he sure as hell isn't going to ramble on about the wonders of radiotherapy.

The patients who are offered curative therapy (i.e. those with a life expectancy of more than ten years with aggressive tumours according to cellular examination), are unfortunately members of the subgroup where impotence, in particular, can be absolutely devastating. Often in the prime of their lives with a healthy and gratifying sex life (and, given the high divorce rates in midlife, not uncommonly living with younger wife number two), they have the most to lose from the complications of surgery.

There are a range of other treatments for prostate cancer including bilateral orchidectomy (Yip, removal of the testicles) and drugs that inhibit production or action of testosterone. These are used for more widespread disease and focus on controlling cancer growth. They are not curative.

So think carefully about screening for prostate cancer. Understand the implications. If you are diagnosed with prostate cancer, obtain multiple medical opinions and include in those opinions an oncologist (medical cancer treatment expert), a radiotherapist, and a surgeon - perhaps in that order.

Remember too, the definition of a cure. Aggressive medical management may be effective in eradicating the cancer but can hardly be regarded as a cure in the true sense.

And me? I am personally not going to subject myself to the screening process. The true value of screening and the ideal treatment of the disease (if any treatment at all is indicated) remain too uncertain at this stage.

- There is currently no evidence that prostate cancer screening improves life expectancy.
- Treatment can produce severe long-term side-effects.
- Be very, very careful and understand the implications clearly before agreeing to screening.

References

1. RANSOHOFF DF, MCNAUGHTON COLLINS M, FOWLER FJ. Why is prostate cancer screening so common when the evidence is so uncertain? A system without negative feedback. *Am J Med* 2002; 113(8): 663-7.

2. SCHRODER FH. Screening for prostate cancer. *Urol Clin North Am* 2003; 30(2): 239-51.

Chapter 20

Colorectal cancer
screening and other gut bits

Cancer of the large bowel (the colon and rectum) is the second commonest cause of cancer-related death in the USA. About 130,200 cases occurred in the US in 2000, and 56,300 deaths were due to the condition. I have an emotional investment in this disease as my mother died from colorectal cancer during that year. Ninety percent of these cancers occur in patients over the age of 50. Colorectal cancer is one of the cancers where we would expect screening to be effective. The cancer usually develops slowly over some years and is preceded by a pre-cancerous stage. The illness starts typically with the development of a benign (i.e.non-cancerous) polyp. The polyp is visible on colonoscopy as a fleshy outgrowth looking something like a mushroom. As the polyp enlarges, the tendency for it to undergo malignant (i.e. cancerous) transformation increases. About 45% of polyps greater than two centimetres in size are cancerous. Usually the polyp-cancer sequence takes five to seven years to develop, but in certain inherited cancer syndromes, evolution to cancer can occur far more rapidly. Because of the slow evolution of the illness and the ability to remove pre-cancerous polyps during colonoscopic examination of the bowel, the opportunities to prevent the illness, or at least to diagnose it at an early curable phase, are exciting.

First of all, let's deal with those conditions that are associated with an exceptionally high risk of developing colorectal cancer. These include:

♦ Familial Adenomatous Polyposis of the colon (FAP) and variants of this condition including attenuated FAP, Gardner's variant and Turcot's variant.

♦ Hereditary Nonpolyposis Colorectal Cancer (HNPCC: also known as Lynch syndrome).

♦   Long-standing inflammatory bowel disease.

♦   Peutz-Jeughers syndrome.

♦   Multiple Juvenile polyposis.

♦   Ureterosigmoidoscopy.

Enough already. Most individuals with these conditions will be well aware that they have the problem or that there is a family history of cancer of the large bowel. These patients should be under the care of a gastroenterologist and undergo screening or other treatment as indicated by the specialist. Inherited colon cancer families usually have several first-degree relatives spanning several generations who have had colon cancer. The cancers tend to occur at a younger age. So if you have a family history of colon cancer occurring at less than 50, or have several first-degree relatives who have had the condition, regard yourself as high risk and see a gastroenterologist. Similarly, patients with ulcerative colitis and Crohn's disease should raise the issue with their doctor if they are not currently participating in a screening program.

OK, what about the rest of us? If you have a single family member who has had colon cancer, your risk is two to three times the average. Most colon cancers, however, seem to be sporadic and related largely to environmental factors, such as a diet high in animal fat, tobacco use, obesity, and perhaps low dietary fibre content. There is general agreement that screening of some sort is indicated. In the average individual (no family history), the American Cancer Society (ACS) recommends annual digital rectal examination starting at age 40. Given the length of the average index finger compared to the length of the average large bowel (1.8 metres), this screening technique is obviously going to miss one hell of a lot of tumours. Accordingly, I find this rationale hard to understand. At the age of 50, the ACS recommends annual testing of stools for occult blood i.e. blood invisible to the naked eye. Several large studies have shown this to statistically reduce the risk of colorectal cancer when undertaken in large populations. Nevertheless, it has several serious limitations. Fifty percent of cancers will be missed, as colon cancer tends to bleed intermittently. Less than 10% of those with a positive test will have an underlying cancer. Another 20% will have one or more polyps.

Unfortunately, everyone with a positive test will need a colonoscopy and that results in a large number of unnecessary investigations. Furthermore, colonoscopy is not an entirely innocuous procedure. There is an awful prep to clean out your bowel, necessitating a sleepless night prior to the procedure. Colonoscopy can be uncomfortable and there is a small risk of complications such as perforation, bleeding or, very rarely, death. And it is expensive. Other screening options include barium enema, flexible sigmoidoscopy (limited to the last 50cm of the large bowel), or the newer technique of virtual colonoscopy. The most accurate test in expert hands is colonoscopy. It has the added advantage of enabling biopsy and polyp removal. At the moment the controversies persist, but I would suggest individuals at average risk either undergo annual digital rectal exam and faecal occult blood screening (as described by the ACS) or a colonoscopy every ten years starting at age 50. If you have one first degree relative who has had colon cancer, colonoscopy every three to five years starting ten years prior to your relative's cancer diagnosis is reasonable.

Gastro-oesophageal reflux disease (GORD) has become more common over the last few decades. Symptoms include, in particular, heartburn and regurgitation. This occasionally is complicated by a condition called Barrett's oesophagus. Barrett's oesophagus has a relatively small risk of leading to cancer of the oesophagus. Screening is not currently proven to be of value in saving lives by detecting early cancer in patients with Barrett's oesophagus and is not universally advocated at this moment in time. If you do have Barrett's oesophagus or longstanding GORD, discuss the issues with your doctor.

- Colon cancer screening options are available and at the very least, faecal occult blood testing should be considered for those at average risk after the age of 50.
- Colonoscopy should be considered at the age of 50 and every ten years thereafter.
- High risk individuals must undergo colonoscopy screening.

References

1. BYERS T, LEVIN B, ROTHENBERGER D, DODD GD, SMITH RA. American Cancer Society guidelines for screening and surveillance for early detection of colorectal polyps and cancer: update 1997. *CA Cancer J Clin* 1997; 47: 154-60.
2. SPECHLER SJ. Screening for Barretts esophagus. *Rev Gastroenterol Disord* 2002; 2 Suppl 2: S25-9.

Chapter 21

Osteoporosis or why are you softening me up like this?

I guess I better say something about osteoporosis as it is preventable, treatable, and is common. It does increase risk of death in the elderly as a consequence of hip fracture, but is more of a problem in reducing QALYs than as a big killer. Osteoporosis is simply defined as weakening of bone, resulting in reduced bone strength and increased risk of fracture. The common sites of fracture are the hip (this has a 50% fatality rate in the very old and frail), the spine (Hey, how come I'm shrinking?), and the wrist. The major victims of osteoporosis are post-menopausal women. This explains why no-one has ever won the Nobel Prize for research into the condition. It has not been a male research priority in the past.

Risk factors include family history, Caucasian background, early menopause, use of corticosteroids (as in arthritis and asthma), low body weight, current smoking, liver disease, personal history of fracture as an adult, alcoholism, inadequate exercise, poor eyesight, general frailty and recurrent falls. Simple preventive measures include stopping smoking, avoiding excessive alcohol, exercising regularly, reducing caffeine intake, and hence, generally having a rather miserable time of it. Adequate calcium intake is important for those at risk and should be in the region of 1200mg daily. Vitamin D supplementation is mandatory for adults. An easy formulation is part of a daily multivitamin supplement and should be about 800 International Units daily.

The Osteoporosis Foundation recommends bone mineral density (BMD) testing in all women aged 60 to 65. The Food and Drug Administration agency is more conservative. Nevertheless, patients at risk should ensure adequate calcium and vitamin D intake and discuss screening options with their healthcare professional. Specific effective therapy is available for established osteoporosis. The most encouraging group of drugs available for specific therapy are the bisphosphonates.

- Screening for osteoporosis is sensible for those at risk.
- Vitamin D and calcium supplementation should be taken for those at risk.
- Effective therapies are available for established disease.

References

1.   COMPSTON JE, COOPER C, KANIS JA. Bone densitometry in practice. *BMJ* 1995; 310: 1507-1510.

Chapter 22

Handguns and rifles in the home
Their role in preventing commanche raids

Finally, a chapter perfect for those 10% of men who read non-fiction books pertaining to personal health and well-being. Sadly, the consequences of widespread and indiscriminate access to guns invariably impact severely on the female of the species. And that is why it is so important for women to read this chapter. To promote changes in the law regarding accessibility to firearms, intelligence and emotional sensitivity are essential. And trust me girls, that isn't going to come from a chemical reaction between testosterone and the male brain. Women need to drive the process.

I have to admit it though folks, I love guns. Yip, I am a real gun nut. It all started with growing up in South Africa. Africa is a vast, sprawling, violent continent, fired by the emotions of its people and the unrivalled majesty of its physical beauty. The rhythms of life and death are as obvious as the seasons. Physical violence is endemic, fuelled by poverty, ignorance, disease, and an aura of hopelessness so pervasive on the continent. Nowhere else in the world is the discrepancy between rich and poor so great. This mix is a recipe for a life that is nasty, brutish and short. Accordingly, the "haves" buy guns to prevent the "have-nots" from attempting involuntary wealth redistribution. The "have-nots" steal or murder to obtain guns in order to convince the "haves" that such involuntary wealth redistribution would be in their best interests. And so it goes. But I digress.

Let me continue about my love affair with weapons. I purchased my first handgun at the age of 18 in the late 1970s. This was the minimum legal age at which one could purchase a firearm in the "old" lily-white apartheid South Africa. Black people were not usually afforded the luxury of obtaining a firearm license. This provided the white population with a considerable advantage in any firefight. My first firearm was a Colt .38 Detective Special. It carried six bullets and was easy to conceal. It provided me with that sense of manhood that is so transparently lacking in most males during late adolescence. I practised my shooting regularly. I cleaned, oiled and caressed the weapon after every outing. I joined shooting clubs and participated in competitions. Being a shooter was a rite of passage to manhood.

Next thing I know, I am drafted into the South African armed forces for two years. This was in the early '80s, where attempts to liberate the country from the apartheid regime were widely regarded by the establishment as part of an elaborate communist plot (but let me reassure you, not by me). As a young doctor, I was given basic training and provided with all the necessities of military life; a FN automatic rifle (Belgian in origin and prone to stoppages), a 9mm Star parabellum pistol, a stethescope, and an all expenses paid trip to Southern Angola. Ammunition for target shooting was available in vast quantities and we blazed away until most of the hair cells in our inner ears were irreversibly kaput. Over the following decade, the love affair continued unabated. I now had three firearms; my trusty Colt .38 Detective Special, a Glock 19 (an exceptional weapon), and a Smith and Wesson .357 Magnum. On one particular occasion I attempted to carry them all concealed in various places on my person, but my spouse refused to let me exit the family home, saying that I resembled Quasimodo. Dirty Harry, where the hell were you when I needed you?

South Africa was becoming increasingly violent at that stage as a consequence of crime and political conflict, and I was by no means heavily armed in relation to the general population. Was I safer with all this weaponry? Were my family more secure? I think not. I always knew this, but was reluctant to retire the armoury. A gun might have protected us if our car broke down in a remote area. Even then I doubt I would have won a firefight, as the opposition were invariably armed to the teeth with AK 47 automatic rifles. And who wants a firefight with your family as the backstop. At home the guns were kept in a secure safe (children lived there) that limited quick access. Owning a firearm in South Africa requires a license that is never provided to those with past criminal convictions. The value of guns to the criminal fraternity is thus enormous and it remains common for people carrying firearms (including the police) to be murdered for their weapons. Similarly, knowledge of a gun safe in a house substantially increases chances of a break-in. Burglary usually involves multiple heavily armed felons forcing their way into properties while families are resident, in order to easily obtain safe combinations and jewellery collections etc. Fatalities are common. It is thus vital to conceal your weapon and ensure your safe is well concealed.

Car hijacking evolved into a hugely successful industry in the '80s and '90s. South Africans have always been obsessed with expensive cars. Cars that cost as much as a small house are much, much easier to steal than robbing a bank. Sophisticated car alarms and immobilising devices have made breaking into vehicles and short-wiring the starter motor an anachronism. Hence the expanding use of carjackers by organised criminal gangs. Car hijacking typically occurs when the occupant has driven out of the family home and exited via the automatic gate. Twenty-foot perimeter walls are useful to carjackers, as they provide excellent concealment. One carjacker approaches from the driver's side and points his weapon at the driver's head. A second carjacker approaches from the rear passenger side and points his weapon at the driver's head. Now even Wyatt Earp would battle to draw his weapon and take out the individual felons before being shot dead. I should also mention that most carjackers are bottom of the car theft food chain. They seldom have much experience with firearms and are frequently very, very jumpy. They tend to have a penchant for shooting first and asking questions later. Carjackers often hang around traffic lights late at night or follow women home from shopping trips etc. Crime statistics in South Africa show that the mortality from a carjacking, provided you don't resist or carry a weapon, is about 1%. That's not too bad i.e. about the same risk as undergoing gallbladder surgery. Carry a weapon or resist, and the mortality rises dramatically, to about 40%. Furthermore, in South Africa if you are shot, it is most commonly with or for your own weapon.

The bottom line is that owning a gun in South Africa increases rather than decreases your risk of death by violence, and South Africa has one of the highest murder rates in the world. I know exactly what the Wyatt Earp wannabees are thinking now - have your weapon at the ready on your lap at all times and approach threatening situations with extreme caution. Well folks that isn't a realistic solution. Hawkers selling everything from fake radios to curios usually frequent traffic stops and traffic lights. When an individual approaches your vehicle it is impossible to distinguish between a hawker and carjacker until it's too late. In the new South Africa (which in my view has the finest constitution in the world, in spite of all these issues), blowing away hawkers is actually a crime. So is waving a gun around whenever anyone approaches your vehicle.

So what's my point? The situation in the US is totally different. You guys are at ongoing risk of attack by Indian warriors. And that is why the right to bear firearms is enshrined in the constitution. A personal armoury is vital. It is the only way to stay safe. And besides, guns can be cool. Man, I know that as well as the next dude. Competitive shooting is really a martial art. Guns are also essential for the national pastime of hunting. It is a little difficult to see how useful a .38 Detective Special or Mac 10 might be in shooting a deer or turkey, but I suppose each to his own.

Anyway, enough of the passion. Let's have a look at the evidence. The commonest method of suicide in both men and women in the US is by handgun. There is even a documented case of a man who shot himself simultaneously in both sides of the head using two handguns. Firearms are responsible for three times the number of suicides than the next leading method. There is data from a wide range of studies (Class II evidence) suggesting a strong relationship between firearms in the home and risk for suicide. You don't have to be a rocket scientist to at least recognise the strong hypothetical case for such an association. Suicide is often an impulsive act. Obviously most seriously depressed people have considered suicide at some time but even in that context the absence of an immediate tool seems to prevent most of these patients from going through with the act. A study in the US showed the introduction of a "cooling-off" period after purchase of a gun of one month before physical ownership could be obtained, substantially decreased the incidence of suicide. What is crucial to note is that the overall incidence of suicide dropped, not simply gun-related suicide. The gun lobbyists suggest that suicidal individuals would have killed themselves by another method anyway, but the evidence does not support this. Easy access to a quick, painless, effective means of suicide substantially increases suicide risk.

Homicide! Arm yourselves folks and increase your risk for homicide, either as perpetrator or victim. Guns are tools designed to kill. Simple as that. Let's get real. Most gun-related homicides, unfortunately, occur among individuals who know each other rather well i.e. family members. You know the story. You and your wife have a few drinks, an argument starts, an ancient affair by one or other party is recalled, things go from bad to worse and kaboom! Someone gets shot. There are a million different scenarios in which this type of tragedy can occur, particularly when fuelled by alcohol or drugs. Keeping a gun in the home unequivocally increases risk for suicide and homicide in the home.

Next come the unintentional shootings. The fascinating aspect of this is that these almost invariably occur as a result of negligence or ignorance about firearm handling and safety. It is common for loaded weapons to be neither locked away nor to have trigger locks. Once a small kid finds the weapon, the chances of inadvertently shooting himself, a family member, a pet, or a friend, escalate dramatically. And that's just the tip of the iceberg. Wait until a suicidal or homicidal adolescent finds the weapon. Whoopee! Next thing we have a suicide, another Columbine massacre, some nut going postal, or a serial sniper.

So what's the bottom line? Guns are dangerous. The USA database researching gun ownership confirms that violent death (accident, suicide or family homicide), is far more likely when there is a gun in the home. The use of a gun in self-defence in the home context is unusual and comprises at most, 4% of firearm-related episodes. In one study, for every occasion that a gun in the home was used for self-defence or a legally justified shooting, there were four unintentional shootings, seven criminal assaults or homicides, and 11 completed or attempted suicides. If one realistically required a firearm for protection (say in the modern South African environment for example), the following would be necessary:

♦ A high standard of training in the safety and use of firearms (police level proficiency).

♦ Compulsory gun safe for storage with either a combination lock or absolute control of the key at all times.

♦ Immediate access to the weapon at all times. A firearm is a tool you hardly ever need, but if you do, then you are going to need it very, very urgently. This effectively means carrying the weapon on your person as a routine, even inside the home if home invasion is a risk.

♦ Formal licensing of weapons.

♦ The absence of weapons in any home with a family member who has a history of depression or other mental illness.

♦ Beware of adolescent access to firearms!

In a civilised society routine access to firearms, particularly handguns and automatic weapons, is crazy. Scenarios like the recent Washington serial sniper case and Columbine will continue to occur. I am amazed that class actions have yet to be bought against gun manufacturers. The National Rifle Association (NRA) is obviously an enormously powerful lobby against any further form of firearms legislation, but new laws restricting firearm access and increasing safety features are inevitable in the long-term. Civil litigation should help drive the process. What the hell is the legal fraternity up to? Surely they are not intimidated!

The real arguments, of course, are not based on rational thought but rather on emotion and passion. I fully acknowledge this. I derived considerable enjoyment from my shooting. There was undoubtedly a time in my life where I would have been an avid supporter of the NRA.

Why then, have I been babbling on against the pro-gun lobby? Simple really. The safety of wider society should take precedence. So, I sold my weapons and emigrated. Call me utilitarian. I can take it.

Incidentally, have you ever seen a dying gunshot victim? Let's choose a soldier who, truth be told, is a special forces operator and, understanding the hazards of sophisticated weaponry in civilian hands, is not a NRA member. Being an expert special services soldier, he well understands that when you go to war you get to play for real. I know that some of my stuff is pure doggerel, but sometimes the impact of poetry is useful to get a message across. Furthermore, there are memories that live with me that I can't erase.

Chest Wound

Flat-backed
Watching a cold and distant moon
Coursing across some stranger's sky
Lifeblood dissipating
Into a soil
That knows nothing
About the loves and laughter
Of youth spent
In a far and foreign place
Of endless summers

OK. No more poetry. After all, the poetry market is pretty limited at the best of times.

Oh, and by the way, death doesn't usually come quietly. The heart stops, blood flow to the brain ceases and a terminal seizure occurs. The contortions, gurgling and twitching can continue for 10-15 minutes.

- Guns are specifically designed to kill.
- The presence of a firearm in the home substantially increases the risk that you or a family member will die by gunshot.

References

1. KELLERMAN AL. Guns and homicide in the home. *NEJM* 1998; 339(13): 928-9.

2. KELLERMAN AL, SOMES G, RIVARA FP, LEE RK, BANTON JG. Injuries and deaths due to firearms in the home. *J Trauma* 1998 45(2): 263-7.

3. KELLERMAN AL, WESTPHAL L, FISCHER L, HARVARD, B. Weapon involvement in home invasion crimes. *JAMA* 1995; 273(22): 1759-62.

4. EILERS R. What physicians can do about firearm violence and prevention. *NEJM* 1994; 91(12): 859-61.

5. CONWELL Y *et al.* Access to firearms and risk for suicide in middle-aged and older adults. *Am J Geriatr Psychiatry* 2002; 10(4): 407-16.

6. GROSSMAN DC, REAY DT, BAKER SA. Self-inflicted and unintentional firearm injuries among children and adolescents: the source of the firearm. *Arch Pediatr Adolesc Med* 1999; 153(8): 875-8.

7. BAILEY JE *et al.* Risk factors for violent death of women in the home. *Arch Intern Med* 1997; 157(7): 777-82.

8. BRENT DA. Firearms and suicide. *Ann N Y Acad Sci* 2001; 932: 225-39.

9. SANGUINO SM *et al.* Handgun safety: what do consumers learn from gun dealers? *Arch Pediatr Adolesc Med* 2002; 156(8): 777-80.

10. GARBARINO J, BRADSHAW CP, VORRASI JA. Mitigating the effects of gun violence on children and youth. *Future Child* 2002; 12(2): 72-85.

11. ISMACH RB *et al.* Unintended shootings in a large metropolitan area: An incident-based analysis. *Ann Emerg Med* 2002; 41(1): 10.

Chapter 23

Road traffic deaths
26 million can't be wrong

Since the invention of the motor vehicle, about 26 million people have been killed in road traffic accidents. These deaths include pedestrian deaths. The absolute numbers are startling and confirm how essential motor transport is, given that it is associated with a significant risk which is nevertheless tolerable to society. It's listed up there among the 12 commonest causes of death.

So what do you expect me to do? Recommend you return to a horse and buggy? Or take advanced driving lessons? Actually, there's not a hell of a lot of advice I can give that is not known to road users. Don't drive drunk or drugged or stupidly. Don't drive when fatigued. If you keep falling asleep when your in-laws visit, you may be suffering from sleep apnoea (OK I agree, boredom is more likely) and should have a medical check. Sleep apnoea increases your risk for a road traffic accident.

Have your car serviced regularly. Wear your seatbelt. Try to avoid road rage. Do not make rude or insulting gestures to other road users, particularly those larger than you. Do not use cell phones while driving. There is class I evidence that such use doubles the risk of a traffic accident. Interestingly, many pedestrian fatalities are found to be drunk at the time of the accident. So remember, sometimes you might not just be too drunk to drive, but also too drunk to walk. The risk of causing a motor vehicle accident is five times greater for males under the age of 25. Why am I not surprised? Because I too was once a male under the age of 25.

References

1. BUNN F *et al*. Area-wide traffic calming for preventing traffic-related injuries. *Cochrane Database Syst Rev* 2003; (1): CD003110. Review.
2. O'NEILL B, MOHAN D. Reducing motor vehicle crashes and deaths in newly motorising countries. *BMJ* 2002; 324(7346): 1142-5.
3. PETRIDOU E, MOUSTAKI M. Human factors in the causation of road traffic crashes. *Eur J Epidemiol* 2000; 16(9): 819-26.

Chapter 24

Does viagra cure depression?

How do we differentiate between anxiety and panic in the middle-aged male of the species? Simple. Anxiety is the emotion experienced the first time you can't get it up a second time. Panic ensues the second time you can't get it up a first time. Funny, ha ha.

Actually no. Let me say it again. Human beings are physical, mental, intellectual, emotional, spiritual and sexual beings. OK, so does Viagra cure depression? Well, it depends. You are a frustrated widow of 72. You win the Lotto and the prize is a Tom Cruise look-alike for the weekend. And try as he might, he cannot perform. Not even once. Are you going to feel depressed? Well of course you are going to feel a bit down. This kind of opportunity seldom occurs in a single lifetime. So what's to do? The reality is that most causes of impotence in males over the age of 40 are related to the use of drugs for treatment of other conditions or to vascular disease, which interferes with blood flow to the penis. Other rarer conditions such as hormone deficiencies are less common. Does therapy help? Of course it can help. The options are Viagra (sildenafil) or newer similar agents such as Cialis (tadalafil) that should impact significantly on the market within the next year or two, injections into the penis, and insertion of drugs into the penile orifice. Surgical options include insertion of a permanent penile prothesis. Sexual activity continuing into old age is the norm, not some strange aberration practised by a perverted minority. Every new generation thinks that they invented sex. Patronising the elderly regarding sexual matters is insulting and stupid.

Keep at it folks, as long as it is not coercive, exploitative or potentially harmful. Swinging from the chandelier is best avoided if you suffer from advanced osteoporosis, for example. Nevertheless, arousal takes a trifle longer, erotic material is frequently useful and subdued lighting may not be a bad idea. Help is available for those with problems. Let me emphasise again that most ongoing impotence is not psychological in origin. In my experience, satisfactory sexual relationships are a vital cornerstone of marriage and other long-term relationships. Furthermore, a study has confirmed the efficacy of Viagra in alleviating depression in previously impotent men. Sexual drive is probably the strongest basic instinctive drive. That makes sense given the fact that it is essential for the propagation and hence survival of the species. Failure to satisfy sexual needs almost invariably leads to significant physical and emotional distress.

The development of Viagra and similar drugs is likely to have a dramatic effect on wildlife conservation. We finally have a group of drugs that really improve sexual potency. In the past, the drugs recommended almost always relied on a strong placebo effect. Whenever placebo is a major player, marketing becomes critical. Rhino horn is a classic example of this. The African rhinoceros is a large, powerful, horny beast with poor eyesight and limited intelligence. Remind you of anyone? Anyway, for some strange reason, the human male identifies strongly with both the rhino and rhino horn. Rhino horn became a real favourite in Asia as a result of the belief that it improves sexual potency. The consequences have been catastrophic and the rhino remains on the endangered list. Poaching is an ongoing problem. The money recouped from selling a single rhino horn can feed an impoverished family for several years. And this is where Viagra comes in. The treatment actually works. This is usually patently obvious to the user. Rhino horn comes a distant second. Modern medicine may just be in a position to save the rhino from extinction. Who said natural is always better? Furthermore, some shady individuals promoting herbal remedies for impotence have been sneaking a touch of Viagra into these preparations. This is all very well, but Viagra should not be used in patients taking nitrates (drugs used in the treatment of angina). Interactions have been fatal. When using herbal remedies you need to be careful. They are not necessarily innocuous. I elaborate further in the chapter on alternative therapies and complementary medicine.

- Impotence has potentially serious implications related to quality of life and sexual harmony.
- Effective treatment is now available for the vast majority of those afflicted.
- Impotence carries a stigma that results in under-utilisation of effective treatments.

References

1.   NURNBERG HG *et al.* Treatment of antidepressant-associated sexual dysfunction with sildenafil: a randomised controlled trial. *JAMA* 2003; 289(1): 56-64.

Chapter 25

Malignant melanoma *et al*

Greetings to all my distant relatives and friends with a dash of Celtic blood. We are the tribes who have evolved to live in the northern hemisphere, typically in wintry climes with limited sunlight exposure. How does the combination of red hair, blue eyes, and a tendency to turn a particularly ridiculous roasted pink confer a survival advantage in the miserable weather of the north? As you probably know, the skin synthesises vitamin D, which is essential for calcium absorption and bone growth and integrity. Adequate blood levels of calcium are essential for muscle and nerve function and a large range of chemical reactions essential for life. Increased skin pigmentation interferes with ultraviolet light absorption by the skin and hence impairs the ability of the skin to produce vitamin D. As a result, minimal skin pigmentation confers a survival advantage in cold wintry lands. Also, black skin functions rather badly as a form of camouflage against a snowy backdrop. Isn't evolution wonderful? Well, not always. Living in a cold and miserable environment sucks. As a result, loads of pallid Europeans have migrated to warm and sunny environments in the southern hemisphere. This does, of course, have a downside. Our pink skin is poorly designed to prevent damage from excess sunlight exposure. Eighty percent of our sunlight exposure occurs before the age of 21. Sun-induced skin damage dramatically increases the risk for skin cancer, both melanoma and squamous skin cancer. Melanoma is by far the more deadly cancer. It is asymptomatic in the early stages but can be diagnosed by careful examination under magnification by an expert. Early signs of malignancy in a mole include an increase in size, irregularity in shape, and increasing or variable pigmentation. Melanoma is curable if diagnosed early. Spread beyond the primary site is almost invariably fatal. Annual detailed skin examination for high-risk patients (red or fair hair, turning bright red on trivial sun exposure, blue or green eyes etc.) who live in sunny environments, is strongly recommended. Minimising harmful UV light exposure, using hats, sunscreens, and appropriate clothing is obviously important, but many of us grew up at a time when tanning was cool and half the point of going to the beach. Watching young and otherwise healthy people dying from melanoma is an absolute tragedy, particularly in view of our ability to cure this condition, if diagnosed early.

Squamous cell cancer develops considerably more slowly, and has usually evolved over a period of many years by the time it reaches an incurable stage. Nevertheless, skin lesions that persist, enlarge or fail to heal, need medical evaluation. So get your moles checked out folks; it could save your life. And besides, doctors need the money. Medical insurance premiums are going through the roof.

Ultraviolet light causes premature skin aging in fair skinned individuals as well and the long-term cosmetic disadvantages of tanning should not be underestimated.

- None of us are bullet-proof.
- If you are red-haired, blond, blue-eyed or burn really easily on sun exposure, you are at increased risk of a variety of skin cancers.
- High-risk groups should be checked out once a year.

Chapter 26
Infections

I need to say a few words about infections. It is rare for infection to be the primary cause of death in economically developed countries, except in the elderly, patients with serious pre-existing illness, some patients with long-standing viral hepatitis B or C, and AIDS patients. Death from pneumonia, for example, is usually the *coup de grace* in an elderly individual with multiple other illnesses (in the pre-antibiotic era, pneumonia was often called the old man's friend). Death from AIDS is becoming less common with ongoing improvements in therapy. Further improvements in management are likely to redefine AIDS as a long-standing illness with limited impact on mortality. Nevertheless, the recent emergence of the Severe Acute Respiratory Syndrome (SARS), shows just how rapidly new viral illnesses, or new strains of traditional viruses, such as the flu virus, can disseminate throughout the world, simply because of the speed and volume of modern national and international travel.

All infectious organisms undergo mutations (changes) from time to time during reproduction. There is nothing really remarkable about this. All that really happens is that the copying of the genetic blueprint (DNA or RNA) is occasionally mucked up. There is a wide range of mechanisms in place to correct such errors. These include so-called mismatch repair genes and molecular chaperones. Of course, like most things in life, the system sometimes fails. Most of the mutations, i.e. changes in the genetic script as a result of said muck up, are nonsense mutations and produce a defective gene that doesn't work, resulting in a non-viable or defective organism. One in a million of these errors, however, might just produce a gene that codes not only for a product that works, but also provides the new mutant with a survival advantage. This is how the AIDS and SARS viruses no doubt evolved. The new virus might also have acquired the ability to jump from one species to another. The AIDS virus made the quantum leap from chimpanzee (where it seemed to be relatively harmless to the host) to man, as a result of the consumption of chimpanzee meat in

Central and West Africa. It is thought that a butcher probably injured himself and contaminated the wound with chimp blood during the butchering process. Add a touch of promiscuity and the advantages of international travel at the speed of sound, and the next thing you know, thirty-five million people have the illness. This is why the SARS epidemic has created such emotional and economic pandemonium, relative to the current risk of acquiring and dying from the illness. We remain uncertain of the containability and the long-term impact of the virus. New strains of flu regularly make the jump from poultry to man. Mutations in the AIDS virus have markedly increased the difficulty in producing an effective vaccine against this agent.

SARS is caused by a brand new strain of coronavirus. The disease has a mortality rate of about 5%. Currently no vaccine, specific treatment, or perfect diagnostic test, exists. The worldwide co-operation in isolating and identifying this virus has been remarkable, and, at the time of writing, it appears that a potential worldwide pandemic has been averted by appropriate preventive measures, including isolation and quarantine of patients.

In medieval Europe the spread of plague and the decimation of the population occurred in the context of a medical knowledge base that wasn't even aware that microbes, such as bacteria and viruses, existed at all. Popular theories to explain the dreadful epidemic at that time included mysterious vapours from a recent eruption of Mount Vesuvius and Divine punishment for a host of human sins. Plague had been carried to Europe from the Far East where it was endemic amongst the human and rodent community. Even in the absence of antibiotic therapy, better understanding of the nature of infectious disease clearly would have enabled appropriate measures to be taken and, hence, containment of the epidemic. I should perhaps mention that some of today's alternative remedies were in wide use as the standard of medical care at that time.

Bacteria mutate similarly to viruses, which explains the need for more rational use of antibiotics and the ongoing requirement for newer and more powerful drugs. Drug-resistant bacterial mutants remain a significant problem in the management of infectious diseases. In spite of these caveats, the prevention and treatment of much infectious disease has undoubtedly been one of the major triumphs of modern medical science.

The situation in the developing world is much different. Death from infections is a major cause of mortality. Diarrhoeal illness, that is no more than a minor irritation in healthy first world children, is a major cause of death in third worlders. AIDS, tuberculosis, parasitic illnesses, malaria, cholera, typhoid and a range of diseases almost consigned to the pages of medical history in the developed world, continue to decimate populations in the developing world. Poverty, denial, corruption, and ignorance exacerbate the problem. The consequences are pretty damned tragic, and on a scale too big for most westerners to conceptualise. For example, the incidence of HIV in Botswana is 39%. And I mean 39% of the entire population. Conceptualise that if you can. The implications are horrific, particularly given the fact that most of the HIV positive people are from the productive, young adult population. Furthermore, there is no access to any anti-HIV drugs whatsoever. AIDS is likely to depopulate Africa and cause death and suffering on a scale similar to the plague in medieval Europe. As Stalin said, "One death is a tragedy, a million deaths are just a statistic."

While walking with my young children in downtown Johannesburg a few years back (and armed to the teeth, needless to say), I was party to an incident that brought home to me the lack of insight of us first-worlders (from a very young age) into the great and ever widening divide between the first and third worlds.

Glue Sniffer

Once we met a street child
Emaciated and sick
He had never eaten broccoli
My children stared into his empty eyes
And thought 'God, he's lucky.'

OK, OK, OK. No more poems. I promise.

What are your individual risks for serious infections? In the first world the biggies to avoid are hepatitis B, hepatitis C, and AIDS. All three illnesses are transmitted much in the same way. Intravenous drug abuse, tattooing, and sexual intercourse spread these damn viruses. Hepatitis B is avoidable by vaccination and should be considered for those whose lifestyle (or whose partner's lifestyle) places them at risk. The wide dissemination of information regarding minimisation of AIDS risk makes any further discussion on this topic superfluous. Treatment for hepatitis B and C is available but cure is by no means guaranteed and at this moment in time, prophylaxis remains very important.

By the way, take your annual flu shots, particularly if you are older or have any chronic (i.e. long-standing) illness. The use of a vaccine against pneumococcal infection (the big mamma of pneumonias), should also be considered at five yearly intervals for the same reason. If you have any chronic illnesses, it is extremely important to see your doctor immediately if you present with any symptoms of an infection. These include symptoms of the common cold or flu. Chronic diseases, such as heart disease, emphysema, and kidney disease, substantially increase the risks of any infective illness and require prompt, appropriate therapy. Older patients and those with chronic ailments should consult with their physician or an expert in travel medicine prior to overseas travel so that appropriate advice and vaccinations can be administered as required.

- Those of us with long-standing underlying illnesses are at increased risk of complications if they develop an infection.
- If you are high risk, ensure that you have your vaccines and present promptly to your doctor if you develop symptoms of either an infection or other unusual symptoms.
- High-risk behaviours are at risk of fatal consequences.

References

1. ZUCKERMAN JN, ZUCKERMAN AJ. Current topics in hepatitis B. *J Infect* 2000; 41(2): 130-6.
2. LANVANCHY D, GAVINIO P. Hepatitis C. *Can J Gastroenterol* 2000; 14 Suppl B: 67B-76B.
3. LIANG TJ *et al.* Pathogenesis, natural history, treatment and prevention of hepatitis C. *Ann Intern Med* 2000; 132(4): 296-305.
4. SEALE C. Changing patterns of death and dying. *Soc Sci Med* 2000; 51(6): 917-30.

Chapter 27
Spiritual belief

What the hell has this got to do with a long and healthy life? It's just a statistic folks, and I have no intention of proselytising. People with religious faith (no specific faith) seem to live a few years longer. Admittedly, there are exceptions as in the Middle East currently. Obviously there may be confounding factors that make this association spurious. After all, a highly religious individual is less likely to be a mainlining drug addict, a sex worker, or the victim of a drive-by shooting. It may just be, however, that the optimism, comfort, hope and camaraderie that religion provides reduces the stresses that pre-dispose to impaired immunity and heart attack.

Not big on religion? Try this trick. Sponsor an underprivileged child from a third world nation. The child must be of a different race group, gender and religion to you. You can make a difference, and using this counter-intuitive approach to sponsorship, your emotional perspective might change. This might just confer the spiritual advantage of increasing life expectancy and, dare I say it, should be tax deductible.

And here's another thing. Married people live longer. Now I know that statistics can lie and that some will maintain it just feels longer, but believe me, this is true. The survival advantage occurs particularly in elderly married men. I don't think we need to call in the local rocket scientist to find out why. Men tend to neglect things like regular meals, household chores, taking medications and washing their underwear. An interesting study revealed that widowers consume far more alcohol than married men. This was initially believed to be due to loneliness and depression. Further research however, revealed that they drink more because they are allowed to! So multiple factors undoubtedly contribute to the survival advantage of married men. The information on widows is still awaited - apparently many are having too much fun to respond to research queries.

References

1. MUELLER PS *et al*. Religious involvement, spirituality, and medicine: implications for clinical practice. *Mayo Clin Proc* 2001; 76(12): 1189-91.

Chapter 28

Doc why am I not on ....?

Just a brief checklist of basic drugs that are strongly recommended as part of the standard medication regimen for most patients with the following conditions (assuming of course that there are no contra-indications):

♦ Heart attack survivors/angina sufferers: low-dose aspirin; beta-blocker therapy; a statin; an ACE inhibitor.

♦ Atrial fibrillation: coumarin.

♦ Hypertension: blood pressure control below 140/85; check other risk factors and consider aspirin prophylaxis.

♦ Stroke survivors: low-dose aspirin (unless the stroke was caused by a primary bleed into the brain); a statin; an ACE inhibitor together with indapamide; optimise blood pressure control.

♦ Chronic bronchitis and emphysema: an optimal smoking cessation program (tough shit man); annual flu shot; a pneumococcal vaccination: low-dose oxygen for certain subgroups. Unfortunately, screening programs for lung cancer have not improved survival rates.

♦ Depression: drug therapy; referral to a psychiatrist; maintenance drug therapy.

♦ Diabetes mellitus: a statin; an ACE inhibitor; low-dose aspirin; blood pressure control less than 130/80.

♦ Osteoporosis: vitamin D, calcium, bisphosphonates such as alendronate and risedronate. The role of HRT is currently controversial in light of the recent research results discussed in the chapter on HRT.

Please note that other agents will clearly be necessary for most of these conditions. Take your checklist along to your health professional.

References

1. ACC/AHC. Guideline update for the management of patients with chronic stable angina pectoris. Report of the American College of Cardiology/American Heart Association 2002; 41:1.

2. GIBBONS RJ *et al.* ACC/AHA. 2002 Guideline update for the management of patients with chronic stable angina - Summary Article. *Circulation* 2003; 107: 149-158.

Chapter 29

Potentially serious warning symptoms

This book is essentially about avoiding illness, but recognition of symptoms early is important in minimising your risk of untimely demise.

For cancer these symptoms include:

♦ Unexplained weight loss.

♦ Persistent unexplained pain.

♦ Visible blood in the stools (called haematochezia).

♦ Unexplained change in bowel habit.

♦ Enlargement, change in shape or colour of moles.

♦ Non-healing skin lesions.

♦ Coughing up blood (haemoptysis).

♦ Blood in the urine (haematuria).

♦ Unexplained vaginal bleeding or discharge.

♦ Difficulty in swallowing.

♦ Persistent unexplained hoarseness.

Before you run screaming to your doctor, remember that many other conditions can cause these symptoms. Nevertheless, if you are experiencing any of the above symptoms, it is sensible to be checked out sooner rather than later.

Symptoms of ischaemic heart disease include the following:

♦ Chest tightness or heaviness typically precipitated or aggravated by exertion, although it can occur at rest. The pain or discomfort may radiate to the throat, arms, jaw, back or upper abdomen, or be experienced only at these sites. Associated symptoms include nausea, vomiting and sweating.

♦ Unexplained shortness of breath on exertion or at rest.

♦ Less obvious symptoms include bouts of light-headedness, fainting and palpitations.

Once again, other explanations are possible, but a physician must assess symptoms suspicious of heart disease, urgently.

For stroke, the possible symptoms include:

♦ Weakness or numbness on one or other side of the body.

♦ Headache of abrupt onset particularly if associated with focal symptoms of weakness, numbness or some other functional loss.

♦ Speech disturbance or loss of comprehension.

♦ Sudden loss of vision even if recovery occurs within minutes.

♦ Abrupt onset of confusion.

♦ Vertigo, nausea, vomiting.

♦ Disorientation.

For stroke, emergency therapy is now available which may improve outcome.

These lists are not exhaustive but should be of some practical help.

Chapter 30

Touching on the other
delights of the metabolic syndrome

No, you are not boring.

I have sleep apnoea.

OK. You are eating more than your body needs. In fact, you have been eating more than your body needs for some time. The old bod is hoarding all this surplus energy. It remembers the famine of 50,004 B.C. only too well. You start accumulating fat. Fat gets packed into fat cells throughout the body, including head, neck, chest, heart, thoracic cavity, abdomen and limbs. I have discussed most of the consequences in some detail. It would be remiss however, to ignore all the delights of the metabolic syndrome.

Sleep apnoea is very topical at the moment. The basic mechanism is simple. With increasing body weight, fat accumulates in the neck and narrows the pharyngeal (throat) cavity.

With age, tone in the neck muscles diminishes. Sleep reduces the tone further. When we breathe in, the reduction in the pressure in the chest draws air into the lungs. This negative airway pressure during inspiration causes the throat cavity to narrow. The combination of a fat neck, poor muscle tone, and sleep can cause obstruction to the airway. The sleeper struggles to breathe, resulting in arousal and disruption to normal sleeping patterns. These arousals do not usually wake the patient. Nevertheless, frequent apnoeas (short-lived episodes of airway obstruction) disrupt normal sleeping rhythms sufficiently to leave the patient in a state of chronic daytime exhaustion. The tendency to dose off during the day becomes overwhelming. The diagnosis of sleep apnoea is suggested in an overweight individual with a long history of snoring and excessive daytime sleepiness. Patients suffering from sleep apnoea have double the normal risk of motor vehicle accidents. Hypertension is more common in these individuals, as are the other risks of the metabolic syndrome. Chronic snoring increases the risk for being beaten to death by an enraged spouse (personal communication from my spouse). Falling asleep while your spouse is describing an exciting event during their day can also have detrimental consequences. By the way, telling women that they snore should be done sensitively, gentlemen. It is seldom regarded as a compliment.

The ideal treatment is weight loss. Given the high failure rates of diet alone, additional options are available. There are a number of oral devices available to advance the lower jaw a few centimetres. This reduces the risk of pharyngeal obstruction during sleep. It also makes you look like a Cro-Magnon. These devices can cause jaw pain and tolerance is variable. Masks that maintain a higher air pressure during inspiration, thereby decreasing the risk of pharyngeal obstruction, are more popular and probably more effective. Both oral and nasal masks are available. They are known in the medical lexicon as CPAP masks. CPAP is an acronym for continuous positive airway pressure. They can be uncomfortable to use and are noisy. In my experience, patients seldom adhere to any intervention unless daytime symptoms are severe and the benefits dramatic. The ideal approach for obese patients is weight loss, as the wider implications of obesity are not addressed by these mechanical interventions.

The polycystic ovarian syndrome is characterised by obesity, hirsutism, infertility and menstrual irregularities. The exact mechanisms involved in causing this problem are unclear, but it is thought that obesity results in increased androgen production. Androgen accumulates in fat tissue and is converted to oestrogen. This results in complex changes in hormone regulation resulting in subtle signs of masculinization i.e. a beard and whiskers, erratic periods and infertility. Treatment depends on whether the beard and whiskers or infertility are priorities at that particular time, and includes oral contraceptives, anti-androgens and fertility drugs. Obviously, weight loss would be strongly advisable, but the limitations of this approach as an isolated therapeutic option have been discussed in detail in earlier chapters.

Fatty liver (hepatic steatosis) results from abnormal fat accumulation in the liver. Causes include excess alcohol consumption, a range of medications, diabetes mellitus, high blood fats, and obesity. NASH (non-alcoholic steatohepatitis) is the acronym given to a condition of fatty liver associated with varying degrees of liver inflammation in the absence of alcohol abuse. Most patients with obesity have a fatty liver but do not develop serious liver disease. A small percentage does develop NASH however. This can progress to cirrhosis i.e. irreversible liver damage. Reasons why this is so are uncertain. It is recognised that fatty acids can increase the metabolic stress placed on the liver and lead to free radical-induced liver damage. Furthermore, fat-soluble toxins can accumulate in a fatty liver. Both these factors probably contribute to the liver damage. It is also important to recognise that diseases work additively to bump you off. If you are obese, drink too much, and have hepatitis C, then you are far more likely to develop cirrhosis than if you are simply obese. The cure to fatty liver secondary to obesity, is weight loss. Isn't life a bitch? NASH has only been recognised as a clinical entity for about two decades. It was not a common condition in our skinnier forbears.

Osteoarthritis is characterised by joint damage largely secondary to wear and tear. If you load any joint excessively for long enough, wear and tear is inevitable. No rocket science here. Our joints were not designed for large, heavy, globular bodies and our hips and knees are disintegrating slowly under the load. The fact that we are living longer, obviously contributes to long-term stress on joints and bones and is undoubtedly an important contributory factor to osteoarthritis. Gout is also more common in patients with the metabolic syndrome. Good drugs are available to prevent recurrent gout.

Hip replacements have been a great success. Knee replacements don't last as long, unfortunately. Still, the technology is advancing, so ongoing improvements in the durability of knee replacements can be anticipated in the future.

- The metabolic syndrome is the shortest route to long-term disability and premature death. Use all the tools provided in this book to prevent the problem. Pompous and self-righteous medical advice to lose weight is unlikely to help without additional support and treatment of the potential complications of the syndrome.

References

1. LATTIMORE JD *et al.* Obstructive sleep apnoea and cardiovascular disease. *J Am Coll Cardiol* 2003; 41(9): 1429-3.
2. NEUSCHWANDER-TETRI BA, CALDWELL SH. Nonalcoholic steatohepatitis: summary of an AASI Single Topic Conference. *Hepatology* 2003; 37(5): 1202-19.
3. CAMPBELL I. The obesity epidemic: can we turn the tide. *Heart* 2003; 89 Suppl 2: ii22-4; discussion ii35-7.

Chapter 31

Life partners to avoid

A final word. Avoid lovers who have failed multiple anger management courses. Avoid those who need supervised administration of anti-psychotic medication. Avoid those with a lifetime history of fire setting, bed-wetting and cruelty to animals. Avoid life partners who you first met in a sexually transmitted disease clinic. Avoid old men who are looking for a nurse and housekeeper rather than a lover. Never, ever, shack up with anyone who has more personal problems than you.

And then lighten up and have fun - life isn't a rehearsal. And if indicated (after a discussion with your doctor), take the therapies that have been recommended, including the diets. They work. I promise.

Glossary

Allergic alveolitis An inflammation of the lung tissue excluding the bronchial tubes and due to an allergy.

Amyloid deposits Abnormal deposits of a protein called amyloid.

Anaemia A reduction in oxygen-carrying capacity of the blood as a result of a decrease in the number of red cells produces anaemia.

Artery Blood vessel that conveys blood from the heart to the tissues of the body.

Atherosclerosis Fatty plaques containing cholesterol, fat and smooth muscle cells that accumulate within the intima (internal lining) of arteries. If these rupture into the cavity of the artery, blood clots develop in the ruptured area. These can produce occlusion of the lumen (canal) of the artery and cut off blood supply.

Cancer A tumour (growth) that is composed of cells which have a tendency to reproduce and spread in an uncontrolled way. Cancers are commonly curable in the early stages of the disease process.

Cell The smallest living unit that in large numbers make up the tissues and organs of the body.

Chronic bronchitis Permanent damage to the airways of the lungs, usually as a result of cigarette smoking. The symptoms include cough productive of sputum for more than three months of the year for at least two successive years.

Diverticulosis A condition of abnormal outpouchings of the colon associated with muscular thickening of the wall. Caused by inadequate fibre in the diet. Usually asymptomatic but can lead to problems of infection, obstruction or bleeding.

Drug Any chemical compound that may be administered to humans or animals in the diagnosis, treatment or prevention of disease or other abnormal condition.

Emphysema Permanent lung damage as a result of tissue destruction, usually secondary to cigarette smoking. Usually associated with chronic bronchitis.

FDA Food and Drug Administration. The US body that controls registration of medications, medical devices and foodstuffs. The URL is: http://www.fda.gov/.

Hepatitis Liver inflammation often due to infection.

Herb Any leafy plant without a woody stem, particularly one that is used as a home remedy or flavouring.

HIV Human Immunodeficiency Virus

HRT Hormone replacement therapy - typically used in the context of replacing the female hormone, oestrogen (with or without progestin), after the menopause.

Hypothesis A theory that appears to explain a group of phenomena and forms the basis of experiments or studies, to confirm or refute any true relationship between these phenomena.

Insulin A hormone produced by the pancreas that regulates sugar, fat and protein metabolism. An absolute or relative deficiency of insulin, leads to diabetes mellitus.

Ischaemia Deficiency of blood in a body part, usually due to obstruction or constriction of an artery supplying that part.

Mania An episode of mental illness characterised by abnormal elation, feelings of grandiosity, rapid thought and pressured speech.

Megaloblastic anaemia A reduction in oxygen-carrying capacity of the blood as a result of a reduction in the number of red cells produces anaemia. Megaloblastic anaemia is a consequence of vitamin B12 or folate deficiency.

Metabolism The sum total of all the physical and chemical processes by which a living organism is sustained in a viable state.

Micturition Passing urine i.e. urinating.

Neuritic plaques Flat areas usually due to deposition of an abnormal protein or other substance are known as plaques. Neuritic plaques occur in or within the region of nerve cells, usually in the brain.

Neurofibrillary tangles Abnormal clumps of nerve cell material found within the cell.

Omentum A fold of internal lining (peritoneum) of the abdomen. Can accumulate large amounts of fatty tissue.

Organ A part of the body made up of a variety of tissues, that performs one or more particular functions.

Pernicious anaemia A type of anaemia as a result of failure to absorb vitamin B12 due to long-standing damage to the gastric lining.

Placebo An inactive substance or preparation, given to satisfy the patient's symbolic need for drug therapy, and used in controlled studies to determine the efficacy of medical treatments.

Prophylaxis A medical term for prevention, designed to obfuscate and confuse the public.

Pulmonary hypertension Abnormally high pressure in the arteries that carry blood to the lungs.

Spina bifida A defect in the wall of the spinal canal leading to a protrusion of spinal contents. This in the severest form, leads to bladder and bowel incontinence and lower limb paralysis.

Supplement Additional treatment of any sort.

Tissue An aggregation of similarly specialised cells, united in the performance of a particular function.

Transurethral resection Operation to relieve symptoms of urinary obstruction due to an enlarged prostate gland, that is performed through the penis and thus leaves no external scar.

Unipolar depression The common type of major depressive illness limited to one or more episodes of depression and never associated with episodes of mania.

Unstable angina Angina that is worsening either by becoming more frequent, severe or occurring with less effort: or any angina occurring at rest.

Vein A vessel through which blood passes from various tissues back to the heart.

Ventricular systole The part of the cardiac cycle when the ventricles contract and hence pump blood to the lungs and all other parts of the body.

Vitamin A general term for a number of unrelated organic substances that occur in many foods in small amounts and that are necessary for the normal functioning of the body.